Ten Days to
Optimal Health

A Step-By-Step Guide to Nutritional Therapy
And Colon Cleansing

What People Have Said About the Optimal Health Center's Step-By-Step Guide...

My weight loss is doing well with the program you outlined for me. I have lost 44 pounds and I am continuing with the changes you proposed in your program.

- Al

Not only have the enemas helped the eczema, but they have helped rid me of my bouts with acid reflux, which was keeping me awake several nights per week. In addition, I must add that the headaches, backaches, and constant tired feeling that I had believed to be just part of the aging process are nearly gone after six weeks of your programs of enemas and diet regulation. My appetite has improved to where I don't crave sweets and carbohydrates as prior to the colon flushes. Now I feel like getting out and doing things.

- Carl

I bought the Vit-Ra-Tox kit and I am on my third day of fasting. I am doing intense colonics on a nightly basis. I cannot believe what is coming out of just about every orifice of my body. I have heard about "mucoid plaque" but wasn't sure if it was true or not. Well, take my word for it: it is VERY true!! I wouldn't have believed it unless I saw it.

- John

It appears that cleansing, massage, and other natural therapies are as useful and important for the lower end of the body as they are for other more visible areas, for example one's teeth or hair.

- Deborah

I couldn't wait to tell you how excited I was to take my first high enema using the three quart amber bag I purchased from you last week! I finally was able to take a full three quarts without stopping to refill the smaller "drug store" bag I had been using! I was able to relax and enjoy the full cleanse! I was raised by a mother that believed in the merits of a periodic high enema, given in a gentle and caring way. When I was a child, a two-quart enema was usually sufficient to reach the cecum. But as an adult, the larger volume is required to do the same job. As you might guess, I have always been a believer in enemas and I welcome the service you're providing. Keep up the good work!

- Sheila

I am a recent newcomer to colon therapy, and I believe my experience is similar to many who come seeking relief from a variety of symptoms, including fatigue, joint and muscle pain, bloating, headaches, irritable bowel syndrome, constipation, PMS; the list goes on and on. After six weeks of periodic colon therapy and fasting, combined with a diet rich in vegetable fiber, high-quality protein and essential fatty acids, and low in sugars, carbohydrates and dairy products, I am symptom-free. My energy level has returned to what it was in my early 20s (I am 37), and best of all, I took no drugs to achieve these results.   -Sarah S.

I had trouble with my weight and had struggled with my health and foods for a long time. I heard about Kristina and decided to go and see her. I had colonic hydrotherapy and changed the foods that I ate. I thought I couldn't handle changing what I did, but with Kristina's help, I did. Hurrah! I didn't try to diet; I just followed Kristina's directions. My weight was 154, and now it is 124. I am very happy and feel sooooooooo great that I have a colonic every month now. I encourage others to go and do it. Thanks to Kristina Amelong.

-Barbara K.

It took some effort in the beginning to shift our eating lifestyle (our daughters are still wondering if this is just another diet fad), but once we had a few recipes figured out, things settled down into a smooth routine. I was absolutely dedicated to giving Kristina's recommendations a chance, so I followed her guidance to a "T." I didn't succumb to any food temptations during the month that we worked together. Kristina was a delight to work with. She dealt with topics that I consider to be very personal (primarily related to body waste). The benefits have surpassed my most optimistic expectations. My health goals as I entered into the process were to increase my energy level and clarity of mind. We certainly achieved these goals, as well as the following positive benefits:

- Our entire family is consuming healthier food.
- The color of my skin has shifted from yellowish to pinkish.
- I am no longer taking antacids before bed to avoid acid indigestion (which translates into better sleeping).
- I no longer wake up in the night with phlegm blocking my airway (once again, this helps me sleep more soundly).
- Chronic hip pain that has plagued me for years has almost completely disappeared.
- Lower back pain has been reduced.
- I've lost almost twenty pounds, which enables me to move much more easily (and this wasn't even why I pursued this direction).
- My energy while exercising has increased.

- Christopher G.

Ten Days to Optimal Health

A Step-By-Step Guide to Nutritional Therapy And Colon Cleansing

By Kristina Amelong, CNC, CT

Prosperity Publishing House
Madison, Wisconsin

Ten Days to Optimal Health
A Step-By-Step Guide to Nutritional Therapy
And Colon Cleansing
2nd Edition

Optimal Health Center
For information address:
2158 Atwood Avenue
Madison, Wisconsin
www.optimalhealthnetwork.com

The suggestions in this book are not meant to be a substitute for a careful medical evaluation by your doctor. This book is intended for educational purposes, and the information presented should be used with discretion.

Printed in the United States of America

ISBN: 0-9755899-6-2

*This book is dedicated to the spirit
in all of us that knows how to be healthy.*

Acknowledgments

I want to thank my husband, Tim Cordon who, for many years now, has helped me to heal, to love, and to grow my business. Without him, none of this would have been possible. Second, I want you all to know what a tremendous woman my mother is. She not only put her heart and soul into raising me, but she has stuck by me as I've grown into my full adulthood. She is central in my family's day-to-day life and she has helped me to write this book. Third, I want to give a resounding thanks to my beloved friend, Nina Hasen, who gave me love and tools when I most needed them. Fourth, I want to sing the praises of Janet Gray who has worked with me daily to create the online Optimal Health Network that helps me reach people all over the world. Fifth, I thank my children, Eli, Johannah, Taran, and Rayna for teaching me how to laugh and how to enjoy the little, and not so little, things in life, such as to wrestle and to love music. Additionally, it has been an honor being able to work with and to learn from all my clients, who have made this book possible.

All of the my current life's work was made possible by the hard work that I have done using the tools of the Re-evaluation Counseling Community (www.rc.org/index.html), which helps me to grow spiritually, emotionally, politically and intellectually.

I offer a special thank you to Beth Racette, Laura Marie Thompson, Debbie Zucker, Andrew Shahan, Rachel Diem, Laurel Green, Mike Kingsbury, Billie Kelsey, Doug Wubben, Paulette Salfen, Sharon Hilberer, Karen Bez, Dan Prusaitis, Holly Jorgenson, Amy Anderson, Larry Cohen, Deb Trent, Susan Hutchinson, Mary Hodgson, Harvey Jackins, and Mike Peterson.

In this second edition, I want all of my readers to know that the love and wisdom of Patrice Salter have enriched this book tremendously.

Finally, I give my love to the dedicated and inspired Janet Gray, Austin Ashley, Hallie Ashley, Scott Wilhelm, Kaet Hall, and J.P. Bowman. And a final hats off to my wordsmith, Charles S. Uinal, and to my Technical Editor, Jeff Muendel.

FYI: My training as a colon hydrotherapist and nutritionist is very dear to me. The organizations that provided guidance during my training include:

- The American Association of Nutritional Consultants (www.aanc.net/)

- The International Association of Colon Hydrotherapy (www.i-act.org)

- Healthexcel www.healthexcel.com www.metaboliced.com

- Re-evaluation Counseling, www.rc.org

About the Author

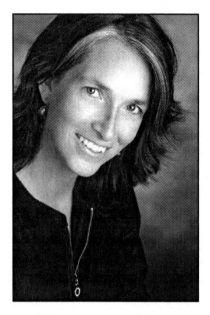

Kristina Amelong is the founder of the Optimal Health Center, the creator of www.optimalhealthnetwork.com, a certified Nutritional Consultant, a Metabolic Typing Advisor, an internationally certified Colon Hydrotherapist, a Re-evaluation Counselor, a wife, a parent of four children, a personal liberation leader, a photographer, a musician, a disabled person recovering from a chronic illness, a world traveler, and a recovering alcoholic.

About This Book

I have spent seven years gathering information for this book and it reflects the evolution in my career as a colon hydrotherapist and nutritional counselor. Readers will discover that the information is organized into chapters, along with the following additions:

Web Addresses

Due to the infomation explosion that arrived with the Internet, readers have an opportunity to research topics that are beyond the scope of this text. To help with this, I have occasionally added Web addresses to many of the book's chapters.

FYI Margin Notes

I've added margin notes to the book simply as "extras." They contain information that I've collected, and the book's wide margins provide a home for these random notes. Don't expect the margin notes to follow the text. Occasionally, they may relate, but that's not intentional; they're intended to be add-ons that relate to the book's overall theme. If you need to refer to the information in the margin notes, you will find the topics in the index.

The World of Natural Therapies and Nutrition

As a health practitioner who is interested in natural therapies and nutrition, I find this is an exciting time to be working with clients. People are waking up and discovering the mistakes they have made. At the same time, practitioners are networking and learning from each other.

I anticipate that my next seven years will be spent learning new developments that I will most likely endeavor to add either to a new edition of this book or to an entirely new one.

Send Me Your Feedback

The Internet is not only an enormous library, but it's also an important communication medium. I would be delighted to hear from readers and learn the following:

FYI: Readers will discover that the nutrition information presented in this book revolves around the work of Weston A. Price. Thanks to Sally Fallon and the Weston A. Price Foundation, Price's work on nutrition is now widely available. The investigations that he did in the early 1930s will have a lasting impact on people all over the world. Price contributed a large volume of work in his lifetime, and most of the details are beyond the scope of this book. To learn about Price's work, go to:

www.westonaprice.org
www.beyondbeg.com
www.price-pottenger.org

FYI: High-quality meats can be hard to find. The following Web sites provide helpful resources:

www.northstarbison.com
www.grass-fedbeef.com
www.eatwild.com
www.ecofish.com

- How you liked this book

- What topics you would like to see covered in my next book

- How you have used the information I've presented

To contact me, log on to the message board on my Web site at www.optimalhealthnetwork.com or send an e-mail message to: Kristina@optimalhealthnetwork.com.

Table of Contents

FYI: Americans are commonly ingesting aspartame, an artificial sweetener that is toxic. To learn about aspartame, go to www.price-pottenger.org/Articles/Aspartame.html.

FYI: Washington, D.C.—based Free Range Graphics has created several Flash movies that champion organically grown food, including:

The Meatrix:
www.themeatrix.com

Store Wars:
www.storewars.com

Chapter 5: What Foods To Avoid and Why

Chapter 6: Five-Day Nutritious-Liquids Fast

Chapter 7: Colon Hydrotherapy

Chapter 8: Therapeutic Enemas

Chapter 9: Implant Recipes

FYI: Free Range Graphics won a 2005 Webby Award for their advocate film called The Meatrix. The film is a Web-based Flash animation that explains how factory farms are ruining communities, the environment, local economies and traditional farm practices. The movie transcript is available in:

• Dutch
• French
• German
• Hebrew
• Hungarian
• Italian
• Japanese
• Portuguese
• Russian
• Spanish
• Swedish
• Turkish

For more details, go to: www.themeatrix.com

FYI: A growing number of consumers care about who is producing their food and how it is raised. Farmers are responding to this development by learning advanced soil management techniques that work without chemicals. For example, they are learning to build a healthy soil environment for organisms such as bacteria and fungi. Just like the "friendly flora" in the human intestinal tract, beneficial soil organisms are the "good guys" that help plants resist the "bad guys" such as diseases, pest insects, and weeds.

Chapter 10: Supportive Case Studies

Introduction

FYI: Remarkably, the history of chocolate sheds light on the oppression that surrounds food consumption: see www.earthsave.org/newsletters/chocolate.htm.

"I write about people, mostly, and the things they contrive to do for, against, or with one another. I write about the likes of liberty, equality, and world peace, on an extremely domestic scale."

-from an essay titled "Knowing our Place"
by Barbara Kingsolver

My name is Kristina. I am a survivor. Today, I am healthy, happy, and proud that after a long battle filled with despair, I am winning! I'd like to share with you my experiences of being sick and my experiences attaining health. I am doing this because I want you to see clearly why I am an expert on the subject of health and healing. Imagine that for many years my days were filled with chronic pain that forced me to be bedridden. My weeks were filled with visiting doctors and specialists who cost a lot of money and still provided no cure. Not only was I facing challenges using modern medicine, but my alternative health path was equally confusing.

My Road to Recovery

First of all, I worked with a naturopathic doctor who had me taking 20-30 different supplements daily and following a strict diet of organic vegetable juice, minimal grains, no meat and vegetable fat. I was also told to do daily colonics, regular fasting and liver cleanses. While on this program, I had my mercury fillings out. This program left me sick in bed for six weeks and with chronic intestinal pain for over five years. I left the guidance of that naturopathic doctor to work with a registered nurse turned health consultant. She again had me taking lots of supplements and following a strict eating program. Even though I diligently followed

FYI: Our current food system is impractical because of the energy (in calories of fossil fuel) that is expended for every calorie of food that is ingested or consumed. Instead of buying food that is shipped thousands of miles, learn to buy food from farmers in the region where you live. To locate farms in your area, go to localharvest.org.

her guidance, my Irritable Bowel Syndrome caused me tremendous pain every single day. After two years of working with her to attain a partial recovery, she discovered that she had cancer and died three weeks later.

Learning to Think for Myself

These tragic experiences have led me on a path that forced me to continue to learn, to figure out how to think for myself, and to heal deeply by digging deep into my pain. My recovery from alcohol and drug use paved the way for this entire experience. I am grateful for the recovery, but it was heartbreaking to have dug myself out of a tremendous amount of emotional pain and addiction, only to be sideswiped by a debilitating illness that I thought would kill me. From these experiences, I have gathered well-researched and broadly applied tools that have worked excellently for me. I know that many of these tools will also work well for you. However, I do encourage you to gather your own tools. My hope for this book is that its contents will assist you in being able to think for yourself about what to look for in a tool that can deeply improve the quality of YOUR life.

Our Body's Healing Ability

Ironically, the many tools that I needed to regain an active, healthy life were readily available. As it turned out, many were packaged within my body, which was just waiting to unleash its marvelous powers. You see, the body is an ingenious, efficient organism, designed to heal and overcome the emotional and physical things that strain it. Unfortunately, we interfere with our body's healing abilities, usually by our lifestyle choices. Through my emotional and physical health struggles, I discovered that systematic laughter, crying, shaking, yawning, and sweating, along with the best possible nutrition, creative exploration, and well-placed detoxification, brought me profound healing from emotional or physical imbalances. This work has brought me to a place of knowing with complete confidence that people have the potential to heal from the mental and physical health struggles we face.

Choosing Optimal Health

Perhaps you have selected this Optimal Health Center plan because you have been feeling run-down or you have symptoms that make your life harder. Whatever the state of your health, chances are it is not quite where you want it to be and you would like some help making improvements. You have made a sound choice because this is my specialty! I am certain that all of us can have better health and even reach our individual Optimal Health level. Optimal Health is the ideal state of our bodies, which allows us increased energy, peace of mind, and a richer life. Unfortunately, this attitude that most of us can choose to set up our lives to enjoy optimal health is not a part of the way that we think as a culture.

My philosophy and ongoing mission are to shift our collective standards of what we mean by health. Optimal Health is more than the, "If it isn't broke, don't fix it," mindset, where after years of ignoring and abusing our bodies (often without realizing it), we try to manage the symptoms that we dutifully accept as, "just part of the aging process"—a mindset in which seventy is considered old and still being alive at eighty is considered lucky. I believe a shift in that paradigm is possible. My ambition is to be old at one hundred and lucky to reach one hundred twenty or more. Would you like twenty to forty extra years of joyful and vigorous living?

Daily Decisions

We need to seize the courage of these convictions and refuse to allow the status quo to wash us down the drain before our time. This mission is big and very appealing; however, through daily decisions, we must take a stand to end the shortsighted view of health that robs us of our vitality.

Let us strive toward our own optimal health. We do this when we realize that to pursue optimal health is to embrace a way of life. Optimal Health doesn't just mean that we take ten different supplements daily, or that we see our doctor for our yearly check-up, or that we are satisfied with taking our cholesterol-lowering medication, or our Prozac. Rather, the path to optimal health is a lifestyle that constantly questions the status quo and holds the

FYI: In 2004, my husband (Tim Cordon) and I bought a farm in Blue Mounds, Wisconsin. I have been following Weston A. Price's principles since 2002 and my family firmly believes in the benefits of raw dairy. We're producing raw goat's milk and free-range eggs for the Madison community. We plan to add cow's milk soon. For details about our farm, see the raw milk page on the Madison WAPF chapter site: www.geocities.com/madison_wapf.

view that when given the proper conditions, the human body can heal, adjust, and function beautifully.

Caring for Our Bodies

Optimal Health is a mindset. It is a way of revering life, allowing rational choice and not convenience, comfort, habit, economy, fear, boredom, or other forces to guide the actions that affect human health. Optimal Health is a path; it is not just a place to reach or a set of skills to attain. It is a journey. It is the daily decision to do things as though your health really matters. When this new lifestyle becomes second nature, we have attained our goal. When we make daily rational choices that promote our health, as naturally as we would choose to remove our hands from a hot oven, then we will love the way we feel and feel more fully the way we love to feel. I believe that if enough of us choose (and yes, it is a choice) to live long, vibrant, and powerful (optimally healthy) lives, our evolutionary trend will shift dramatically in the direction that affirms our human goodness and our ultimate ability to share Earth's bounty for optimal health for all.

Did you know that at this point in history, all of us, unless we are killed by a tragedy, will die of a disease created by the way in which we care for ourselves. This is unacceptable to me. I take issue with the standards that we collectively hold regarding what it means to care for our bodies.

Perhaps this is the time in your path to take stock and to take control of your life and body. You and you alone can make your life the way you want it. You and you alone can pursue your dreams.

My Favorite Radio Shows

Wisconsin Public Radio archives their shows online and listeners can access recordings using RealNetwork's Real-Player that's available as a free download.

The show program notes are also helpful to look up program descriptions, guest names, and topics. To see program notes, go to www.wpr.org/ideas/programnotes.cfm. The following shows are a few of my favorites:

Ode Magazine

To listen to a radio show about how our world is becoming a better place everyday. On the 8:00 p.m. show, of Here on Earth, Jean Feraca learns about "Ode," a magazine dedicated to "things going right." Her guest, Jurriaan Kamp, headed the Economic Desk at the Dutch equivalent of the *New York Times*, but he got tired of all the news of things going wrong. So he and his wife started a magazine dedicated to things "going right"—things you would normally never hear about. It's now also published in the United States.

Catherine Brand and the New Food Pyramid

To learn more about how current research is changing what we collectively believe is a healthy diet, listen to Catherine Brand talk with Sally Fallon about the new food pyramid, created in an effort to curb what some say is an obesity epidemic in America. Time: 9:00 a.m., September, 2, 2004.

Brett Hulsey and Highway Pollution

To learn more about the toxins in your environment, listen to this talk show with Joy Cardin and the lead author, Brett Hulsey, of a report released in July, 2004, that links highway pollution to health risks such as cancer and asthma. This particular episode aired on August 2, 2004 at 6:00 p.m.

FYI: Goat's milk is an excellent source of calium and other nutrients found in cow's milk. It is mostly known for the fact that it can often be used as an alternative for people who are sensitive to cow's milk. Goat's milk is not considered to be a commonly allergenic food. One of the chief reasons for this is that goat's milk is often free of pesticide residues and is not known to contain goitrogens, oxalates, or purines.

FYI: Goats are one of the oldest domesticated animals and the practice of herding goats is thought to be about 10,000 years old. Paintings of goats appear on the walls of ancient caves.

CHAPTER ONE

The Optimal Health Center

FYI: Raw whole milk contains protein, fats and carbohydrates. It is also a very important source of essential nutrients, including:

- Calcium
- Riboflavin
- Phosphorous
- Vitamins A, D, and B12
- Pantothenic acid

"It is through the truthful exercising of the best of human qualities - respect for others, honesty about ourselves, and faith in our ideals - that we come to life in God's eyes."

-Bruce Springsteen, August 5, 2004

My mission for the Center, established in 1998, has always been to help people improve their health in the way that works best for them. To be effective in my recommendations and treatments, I spend much time in discussion with my clients about their lifestyles, eating habits, individual biochemistry, and toxin exposures to understand how to assist them in achieving the goals they have when seeking treatment. It is by means of this conversation that I can recommend a comprehensive treatment plan.

Nutritional Plans, Supplements, and Colon Cleansing

My approach requires that my clients listen to the needs of their own bodies, while adjusting—if not totally changing—their lifestyles. Typically, I provide them with attentive listening, nutritional plans, supplements, and colon and enema hydrotherapy. The program that I most commonly recommend has now become my trademark, *Optimal Health Center Plan.* The *Optimal Health Center Plan* will lead you through well-defined easily followed steps. This plan can help you: build confidence by changing unwanted habits; detoxify your body safely and painlessly, without strenuous juice fasts; get in shape and feel strong within your body; learn what foods are medicinal, so that your body will function better, and feel so much better, that your dietary "shoulds" become active desires to overcome chronic health problems and increase your energy level. Furthermore, it is possible to accomplish this plan very economically within a manageable amount of time!

Your Body's Healing Abilities

I want to highlight the fact that no matter what state of health you are in, you can heal. Your body's healing abilities are intact. If you cut your finger, it will heal. Take a moment to think about that. It is the most important concept that I offer to you: *You Can Heal!* Now continue your journey to great health by reading and by believing in the healing powers of yourself as well as of all those around you.

Frequently Asked Questions

Over the years, many of my clients have asked similar questions. I've created the following "Q & A" so that readers may benefit from seeing the questions others have asked.

Question: *How do people know or recognize the signs that they need to embark on a program of detoxification and therapeutic nutrition?*

Most of us are not aware of our toxicity levels because we become polluted over time and we gradually forget what it feels like to be healthy and energetic. Recently, I was talking to a client whose medical doctor had told him, "There is nothing wrong with you, but there is really nothing right." A sure sign of a body in crisis is a chronic disorder such as Candida albicans, high blood pressure, allergies, Irritable Bowel Syndrome, fibroids, Arthritis, Fibromyalgia or Chronic Fatigue Syndrome. For many of us, frequent bouts of gas, bloating, or feeling generally run-down are signals from our body that we need to detoxify. Even in the absence of specific symptoms, aging itself reduces the body's ability to detoxify. Unfortunately, our world is getting more toxic every day!

Each of us not only accumulates environmental toxins and metabolic wastes year after year, but most of us also lack the necessary nutrients needed by our bodies to truly nourish each and every one of our cells. Most of us take supplements or think we ought to because we are aware of our increased bodily need for nutrients. However, most of us are not aware of the important fat-soluble nutrients that are needed for rebuilding and cleansing each cell and every organ. These fat-soluble nutrients such as vitamin A and D, and Activator X bring needed nutrients into our cells. These nutrients, such as butyrate acid, are the very substances that rebuild our colonic mucosa from the ravages of modern foods. Furthermore, Conjugate Linoleic Acid is the very substance that keeps our immune system strong.

An excellent movie, *Super Size Me*, brings home the sad truth that we are all toxic and need to work through a therapeutic nutritional program such as the *Optimal Health Center* plan.

Question: *What happens when you rebuild and detoxify?*

Above all, you heal. You will feel better. Your body will be able to utilize nutrients, systematically eliminate toxins, rebuild damaged organs, tend to the demands of the cells, and create the needed energy to live daily life and to regenerate health.

In addition, rebuilding and detoxifying can make one feel sick for awhile. Daily living, without adequate nutrients, drives toxins and diseases further into the body, while rebuilding and cleansing permit these wastes and diseases to surface and leave the body via the skin, lymphatic system, lungs, colon, and urinary tract. When people quit smoking, for example, they are very often surprised at the number of colds they get during the months after they have stopped smoking. They thought they were improving their health; and suddenly they find themselves in the midst of a fiery, "healing crisis." A similar situation can occur with a program such as this one. Although this cleansing response occurs for many, not everyone experiences it in the same manner.

Question: *Where is the payoff?*

What you need to know while detoxifying is that any symptoms of ill health are usually not due to a cold virus at all, but are rather the body's way of throwing off accumulated toxins and damaged

FYI: Correctly given, enemas serve as strengthening exercises for the colon. This long tubular muscle is repeatedly and completely filled, inducing it to vigorously exercise while evacuating itself multiple times. The result is a great increase in muscle tone, acceleration of peristalsis and eventually, after several dozens of repetitions, a considerable reduction of transit time.

- *How and When to Be Your Own Doctor*
- Dr. Isabelle A. Moser with Steve Solomon, June, 1997.

cells. The payoff is that within the sweat and phlegm leaving the body are many toxic, carcinogenic residues of PCBs, heavy metals, phenolics or whatever accumulated poisons your body might be carrying. The pay off is the increased energy, mental clarity, and emotional freedom you experience as you follow the plan. For most clients, the dietary and detoxifying program brings better health.

Question: *Why not just fast for detoxification instead of following a 30-day eating program before I fast?*

Fasting using only water, and more recently only vegetable juice and water, is an ancient cornerstone of both physical and spiritual healing. However, due to our current toxic ways of living and the lack of healthy fats in our diet, our bodies don't have enough resources to address the biochemical needs of a fast. The needed nutrient stores in our bodies are too little and the stored toxins in our bodies are too great for a simple fast to address. Today, fasting can easily make people very sick and almost always makes people less healthy.

Fasting does seem to work wonders for a person with an acute illness. During the flu or another sudden illness, our bodies don't desire food; our body's intelligence knows that there is something to get rid of within our digestive tracts. This bodily wisdom works wonders to rid the body of an unwanted virus or bacteria. However, most people need to get rid of environmental toxins and most people also need to rebuild their bodies. You know this if you are feeling chronically run-down, or are sick with Fibromyalgia or another illness.

This cleansing program does have a nutritious liquids fast at the end of a high-nutrient cleansing diet. Both the diet and the fast are based on the principles of eating nutritionally dense and cleansing foods such as raw dairy products and other high-quality fats and proteins, fruits, vegetables, and vegetable juices. Some of this nutritional guidance is new; for instance, the importance of fats in cleansing is poorly understood. Few people, even few alternative health practitioners, know that raw, grass-fed butter is one of our most potent medicinal foods used to detoxify the body:

Therapeutic amounts of raw fats draw toxins out of the cells. Most cleansing programs only carry toxins out of the main circulation and not from deep within each cell, tissue and organ.

Regardless of how healthy you think you are, NEVER fast without significant support: the synthetic chemical toxin load in human fat and muscle today is much greater than that which even a healthy body can handle. In other words, we are all so toxic that even brief fasting is often damaging to the liver and other organs. Thirty years ago this was largely not the case, but it is now. Because of this, my cleansing program has been developed to assist the liver and every cell in the body with the important work of removing toxins and rebuilding the body.

Question: *How do we get toxins out of the places where they are stored?*

Eating therapeutic types and therapeutic amounts of fats and oil is our most effective way to remove toxins. Your body can not fully or easily detoxify without fats and oils within your circulation and deeply integrated into the cells. You need raw fats and oils because lipase, the fat-splitting enzyme, assures that the fats and oils can be taken into the cells. Once the body has the needed fats and oils, the tools of colon cleansing can assure that the toxins are removed and not recirculated throughout the body.

Question: *Why is the book called* Ten Days to Optimal Health?

What makes the Optimal Health Center Plan so effective and easy to use in daily living is that it is based on ten-day segments, where participants practice a new, clinically-based lifestyle ten days at a time. Along with the nutritional protocol, periodical cleansing of the colon of toxins and harmful wastes, through colon hydrotherapy or enemas, is performed every ten days, or less.

Through my clinical work, I have found that the key to a successful program, in which people really change the way they live for long-term results, is to carry out the plan in "Ten Day" segments. Staying focused and on track for at least ten days is an attainable

FYI: In his essay, "The Pleasures of Eating," farmer, author, and poet Wendell Berry says, "A significant part of the pleasure of eating is in one's accurate consciousness of the lives and the world from which food comes."

FYI: The organic agriculture and gardening movement is directly opposed to trans nationals that have industrialized food production. Fifty percent of our food products are controlled by ten giant corporations. The result of this trend has been a downward spiral.

goal for many people. The initial ten-day program is then repeated two additional times and completed with a five-day surprisingly easy and energizing, nutritious-liquid fast. Therefore, in thirty-five days, a new, healthier lifestyle and all the benefits that go with it can be achieved. This approach not only helps people improve their health, but it also raises their confidence, motivation, and staying power. I always tell my clients, "You can do anything for ten days!"

And, I know that most of you want to know at the outset, "Will I need to follow this diet for the rest of my life?" Yes and no. In order to be optimally healthy, you will need to eat nutritious foods and avoid non-nutritious foods. Unfortunately, our world today is full of foods that are not actually nourishing to the human body, but rather meet our communal needs for convenience, relief of loneliness, tradition, and profit. A key component of following a plan is that you learn how truly to understand what foods are healthy for you and what foods are not, so that you can truly think for yourself. What follows are the tools to be able to make the choices for optimal health for many years to come.

FYI: A first step to locate economical sources of natural food might be to network in your region. Collect phone numbers and mailing, e-mail, and Web addresses of everyone you can find who is interested in local agriculture.

CHAPTER TWO

Genetics, the Environment, and Nutrition

"You've heard it before, but it bears repeating: nothing in life is more precious than your health. If you take care of your body not only do you prevent disease and illness and prolong your life, but you also vastly improve the quality of your life."

> Dr. Joseph Mercola
> Dr. Mercola's Total Health Cookbook and
> Program

It is human nature to want to be healthy, vibrant, and energetic. It is human nature to love life from the moment we are born until the moment we die. This innate desire to live well doesn't change as we age. It is clear that people do not want to lose their health, ever. Why, then, are so many people struggling with illness?

The Role of Genetics

To begin our exploration of what influences our health, let us look at what role our genes play. Many people think that our genes fully determine our health, or at least determine the risk of such diseases as heart disease, cancer, and diabetes. What we are certain of is that our genes do have an effect on our aging process. However, the extent to which our health status is inherited is not fully determined.

Certainly genetics play a role in how we age, as well as the diseases that we struggle with. However, our focus on hereditary as the reason for our health woes needs to be examined in the light of our environment.

Linus Pauling's Thoughts on Genetics

In 1949, Linus Pauling, the founding father of molecular biology and author of *Vitamin C and the Common Cold*, *Cancer and Vitamin C*, and *How to Live Longer and Feel Better*, made public his theory that the origin of disease is based on specific changes in genetic materials due to environmental influences, which in turn modify physiological function. In other words, Pauling's theory states that disease is not solely caused by genetics, but rather due to the interaction between an individual's genes and his/her surroundings. Bishop and Waldolz point out in their book, *Genome*, that "aberrant genes do not, in and of themselves, cause disease. By and large their impact on an individual's health is minimal until the person is plunged into a harmful environment..." (Simon and Schuster, New York, 1990). To clarify, it seems that each person's gene pool has the flexibility to express itself with health and longevity, or with illness and degenerative disease, depending on environmental conditions. Unfortunately, we take for granted that when a person's genes do express sickness, or even early death, these diseases are genetic, or destined to occur.

Environmental and Political Factors

It is oppressive the way in which all people are systematically hurt by the belief structures and behaviors of their society. People are forced into decisions that cause their bodies to express disease. We are lied to and made to believe that things that are harmful to health are actually good for us. Why? Because our culture is fixated on profits. In his book, *Natural Cures "They" Don't Want You To Know About*, Kevin Trudeau explains why the United States government, the major food companies and the drug companies systematically promote ideas that may cause people harm.

Our current societal structure prioritizes profit above health. Health is created or destroyed by the way we set up our lives. If we eat well, we tend to be healthier. If we rest deeply and daily, we tend to be healthier. If we are close to other people, we tend to be healthier. If we exercise and spend time outdoors, we tend to be healthier. If we have a rich spiritual life, we tend to be healthier. If we nourish our emotional selves, we tend to be healthier. When all of these activities are combined, most people are going to express health genetically and not disease. Unfortunately, most of us aren't able to pull all of those elements together.

Profitability Before Health

For example, most people don't eat foods that support their optimal health. Most of us don't even know what it means to eat well. Foods and all other ingestible products are produced to have long shelf lives, be conveniently transported, and to be produced with the lowest overhead and the highest profitability. Very few producers of foods, supplements, pharmaceuticals, and other bodily products place health above profitability. Most foods are available primarily for the purpose of the suppliers to make a profit and not for their high nutrient content. Diet ought never be based primarily on the needs of the economy and the way in which the economy encourages people to eat. For example, one in four people in the developed world eat at McDonald's every day.

Limited Access to Quality Food

The average person has very little incentive or education that would lead them to seek out and to choose optimally nutritious food. Most people have limited opportunities to choose the best possible nutrition for their body. How many people have access to organically grown food, high-quality meats, and raw milk from pasture-raised animals? Not many. In our family, we have had to go to great expense to obtain the foods that have assisted my healing, like raw milk and butter and grass-fed meats, even though we live in one of the finest metropolitan areas for organically grown and local food. By understanding how environmental and political factors influence our lives and our cultures, and by healing those scars of oppression, we will be more fully able to eradicate degenerative disease and be optimally healthy.

Nutritional Content of Food

What are the nutritional resources that your body needs in order to be optimally healthy? What is optimal nutrition? Is it possible to practice an optimal diet within a culture that values food for profit over food for health? Through my experiences with healing and working with clients, I have come to believe that we can identify nutritional resources and head ourselves toward optimal nutrition.

FYI: Wendell Berry is a farmer, essayist, novelist, professor of English, and a poet. Far too numerous to list, Berry's works are widely available at bookstores and libraries. *The New York Times* has called Berry the "prophet of rural America." He lives on a farm in Port Royal, Kentucky, where he was born on August 5, 1934. Berry is a strong advocate of family, rural communities, and traditional family farms.

Nutritional researchers have studied cultures whose entire population was much healthier than ours is today. Dr. Weston A. Price analyzed the nutritional content of the diets of our healthiest ancestors to decisively identify foods that create environmental conditions for their bodies to genetically express health and not illness. Looking at our healthiest ancestor's food to determine what foods are therapeutic is turning out to be enormously successful. Well-known nutritional experts Sally Fallon, Dr. Robert Atkins, Donna Gates, Dr. Joseph Mercola, Dr. Andrew Weil, and Dr. Jordan Rubin all share a common theoretical premise: many of the foods our healthiest ancestors ate are now so vital to the well-being of our bodies due to their nutrient content, that they can be considered healing to the body, or medicines.

Principles of Healthy Diets and the Work of Dr. Weston A. Price

What scientific evidence supports the argument that the diets of our ancestors were therapeutic and could assist us to optimal health? To answer this question, I will site the work of Dr. Weston A. Price. Dr. Price, was a prominent dentist and researcher who conducted studies during the 1930s and the 1940s regarding the prevention of tooth decay, gum disease, and orthodontic troubles. Within this context, he sought to understand what makes humans healthy and what allows humans to have perfect teeth—not what pushes people toward illness. His determination to study what makes humans healthy and not what makes humans ill makes his works an excellent source of insight. He details his research methods in his book, *Nutrition and Physical Degeneration*:

> *"Primitive man did not have the same disease pattern as modern man. Primitive man suffered from infectious disease but was almost free of degenerative diseases. Modern man has almost eliminated infectious disease but is suffering from an epidemic of degenerative diseases."*
>
> *- From Health and Healing Wisdom, the Price-Pottenger Nutrition Foundation Journal, Fall 2004, Volume 28, Number 3*

* Weston A. Price first published *Nutrition and Physical Degeneration* in 1939. At that time in history, European writers commonly used the term "primitive racial stocks" to denote indigenous peoples, which I see as offensive and dated. Price uses the term "primitive racial stocks" to mean people, whether European or indigenous, whose diets were untouched by the "foods of commerce." Foods of commerce are foods whose value is seen in terms of profit and not health.

"In my search for the cause of degeneration of the human face and the dental organs I have been unable to find an approach to the problem through the study of affected individuals and diseased tissues. In my two volume work… Dental Infections, Oral and Systemic and…Dental Infection and the Degenerative Diseases, *I reviewed at length the researches that I had conducted to throw light on this problem. The evidence seemed to indicate clearly that the forces that were at work were not to be found in the diseased tissues, but that the undesirable conditions were the result of the absence of something… This strongly indicated the need for finding groups of individuals so physically perfect that they could be used as controls. In order to discover them, I determined to search out primitive racial stocks that were free from the degenerative processes with which we are concerned…"*

He continued, *"To accomplish this it became necessary to locate immune groups which were found readily as isolated remnants of primitive racial stock in different parts of the world. A critical examination of theses groups revealed a high immunity to many of our serious affections so long as they were sufficiently isolated from our modern civilization and living in accordance with the nutritional programs which were directed by the accumulated wisdom of the group."*

The Traditional Diet

Once Dr. Price determined that he needed to study isolated people who appeared to be the healthiest of the peoples on this planet, he spent several years conducting research in his Iowa laboratory before he went into the field. He analyzed the nutrient content of different foods to communicate to the world what nutrients gave health to whole populations of people. As soon as he established his laboratory support, he and his wife set off to learn from the diets of these isolated groups. Every summer, they traveled to

FYI: High-vitamin butter oil and cod liver oil have a synergistic ability to heal that Weston A. Price found puzzling. Sally Fallon explains this in her book *Nourishing Traditions*:

"Dr. Price was often called to the bedsides of dying individuals, when last rites were being administered. He brought with him two things—a bottle of cod liver oil and a bottle of high-vitamin butter oil from cows eating growing grass. He put drops of both under the tongue of the patient—and more often than not the patient revived. He was puzzled by the fact that cod liver oil alone and butter oil alone seldom revived the dying patient—but the two together worked like magic."

remote places and in the end, visited over fourteen tribes, clans, and villages whose members all displayed remarkable freedom from mental, physical, and emotional imbalances. Whether they were investigating the Maori of New Zealand, Irish fishermen, Native Eskimos, the Swiss, Australian Aborigines, African tribes, or Pacific Islanders, they came upon vibrantly healthy people, as long as they were eating traditional diets. This most important discovery was duplicated in all cultures: If the people were eating their traditional foods, they had very little or no tooth decay or physical degeneration elsewhere in the body. Through his continuous research, Dr. Price concluded that tooth decay and degenerative diseases were irretrievably linked and stemmed from the same cause—one's diet. When people cease to eat the traditional, nutrient-rich diet of their native culture and choose instead the "displacing diets of commerce"*, there is a high correlation with illness and disease. It is by eating the simple, basic, nourishing foods indigenous to native culture that individual populations thrive and live long, disease-free lives.

*The "displacing diets of commerce" are diets that are driven by commerce. These foods are available primarily for the purposes of the suppliers to make a profit and not for their high nutrient content. Diet ought never to be based primarily on the needs of the economy. The fact that this has happened is a flaw in our current capitalistic social structure. Dr. Price had the wisdom to strengthen his argument that the body does indeed have requirements for certain nutrients by examining the health status of the same races of people who had changed their dietary ways away from the traditional foods to the foods offered by modern commerce. This gives his work the true gauge of scientific validity. He writes, "In every instance where individuals of the same racial stocks who had lost this isolation and who had adopted the foods and food habits of our modern civilizations were examined, there was an early loss of the high immunity characteristic of the isolated group."

Price's Dietary Principles

Fortunately for us, Dr. Price left detailed records of his research in his landmark work, *Nutrition and Physical Degeneration*. From these records, health professionals and scientists have identified particular foods and particular methods of preparation that are common to each culture. The dietary principles of the fourteen cultures that Weston A. Price studied serve as a guide today in whatever diet we choose. Listed below are eight universal dietary principles that Dr. Price witnessed in every society that he studied. Some aspects of the following principles may not be familiar to you; please know that I will go into further detail on each principle later in the book. The principles that each culture followed are:

1) Ate up to ten times the amount of natural, non-synthetic, vitamin A, vitamin D, and Activator X in the diet as did most people of Dr. Price's day.

2) Never consumed refined or denatured foods including: protein powders, high-fructose corn syrup, hydrogenated oils, white flour, or fruit juice.

3) Used both cooked and raw foods in their meals, especially animal foods.

4) Ate raw foods high in enzyme content: dairy, meat, honey, cultured vegetables and tropical fruits like papaya. Furthermore, consumed lacto-fermented foods and drinks such as kvass, yogurt, and kefir.

5) Always fermented, soaked, sprouted, or naturally leavened their seeds, grains, and nuts.

6) Ate significant quantities (30%-80%) of their total diet in fat. In every case, polyunsaturated fats comprised only 4% or less of the fat in the diet. Omega 6 and omega 3 fats were in a ratio of 1:1, and generous amounts of saturated fats were also eaten.

7) Included unrefined salt in their diets.

8) Used bones for broth.

FYI: As a consumer, you have tremendous purchasing power. As you spend your money on food, think of your purchases as votes that can support fair and environmentally sound practices and veto anything that damages our world.

Now, with the principles of traditional diets in mind, let's explore my basic program, the Optimal Health Center (OHC) plan. The OHC plan is an easy-to-follow, clinically proven, traditionally based, and solidly researched dietary program. Enjoy. And feel free to contact me if you need support. I want you to be successful! And, most importantly, I want you to be able to intelligently choose a healthy diet for yourself.

You ask, "What if I descended from people with very different cultures and eating habits? Do I eat the foods indigenous to where I live now or where my ancestors lived?" I propose that instead of thinking rigidly about the foods your ancestors ate, you take the common dietary factors from each of the healthy cultures that Dr. Price studied to determine your optimal foods. The foremost point to keep in mind is that no matter what 'diet' you choose, you need to eat foods that are rich in specific nutrients in order to be optimally healthy. I will highlight these nutrients as I explain my OHC plan.

CHAPTER THREE

The Optimal Health Center's 10-Day Program

"One of the most helpful things you have said to me is that the world is trying to sell PRODUCTS. It is not interested in my health—it is interested in making money by selling products. Somehow, this has enabled me to turn a deaf ear to all of the layers of persuasive mail I get about how I can be rejuvenated, and revitalized, and re-this, and re-that. I love the fact that you made me aware of this; and, I, of course, marvel that I was not aware of it before."
                                        -an e-mail from a client

The Optimal Health Center's (OHC) program can best be understood in terms of ten-day milestones. The activities included in each of these milestones will be described in detail in the chapters that follow.

Milestone #1: Reaching for a New Normal

Days 1-10
This first milestone includes a colon cleanse and a daily nutrition plan. Together, these provide the intestinal track and the immune system with a fresh start.

Milestone #2: Ten-Day Restart

Days 11-20
This milestone provides an opportunity to assess energy levels, mental alertness, and the presence or absence of pain. A second colon cleanse occurs on Day 10, followed by ten more days of the daily nutrition plan.

Milestone #3: Ten-Day Restart

Days 21-30
Much like milestone #2, this milestone offers an opportunity to assess your progress. A third colon cleanse occurs on Day 20, followed by ten more days of the daily nutrition plan.

Milestone #4 Final Cleanse

Days 31-35
This milestone includes a five-day fasting cleanse that includes three colon cleanses and a gentle conclusion to the five-day fast with support provided by supplements and nutritious-liquids.

OHC Nutrition Program

In the spirit of Dr. Price, I use the nutritional traditions of healthy peoples who lived beyond the reach of modern commerce to lay out a framework of excellent nutrition for you and your family. In addition, within the framework of the OHC plan, I will outline the wisdom that alternative health professionals have acquired while applying natural methods to ourselves, our beloved clients, and our loved ones. For instance, carrying out this plan in segments of ten days is not necessarily a tradition of one of the cultures that Dr. Price studied, nor is eating vegetables or fruits throughout the day. These ideas, which were developed while using foods as medicine for healing, have proved to work well for many people. In this vein, what follows shows what must be done during each ten-day period to achieve the desired results. Each of these steps will be explained in detail in subsequent pages so that you can fully understand the purpose for each. The plan starts with Day One and a colon cleansing session. On this same day, you will begin the Ten-Day Nutritional Program.

Colon Cleansing Options: Hydrotherapy or At-Home Enemas

Colon cleansing is an integral part of this plan. Yet many can be optimally healthy without doing colon cleansing. However, accumulated pockets of fecal matter can dramatically interfere with healing. Accumulated stool can hinder vitamin and mineral absorption, causing nutritional deficiencies. Furthermore, accumulated stool can irritate nerve endings, causing an inflamed bowel, and can release toxins into the bloodstream, causing a poisoning of healthy organs and tissues. Due to my good fortune of being a colon hydrotherapist, I have seen the tremendous amounts of stool that move out of people during subsequent colon cleansing sessions. Many people, but not all, would greatly benefit from regular and gentle cleansing of the colon.

Another benefit of colon cleansing includes caring for yourself in a way that leaves you feeling refreshed, cleansed, light, empty and yet nourished. I have found that because of the resulting feelings from having fully cleared out the entire length of the colon using a gentle treatment of water therapy, most people are able to stick to the challenge of changing their daily habits. For some, this self gift of stick-to-itiveness from colon therapy can make a significant difference in their level of success.

Enemas weren't discussed in Dr. Price's text. Does this mean that tradition-oriented people didn't need or use the added tool of colon cleansing for health? I don't know. However, there are many historical examples of people using enemas to benefit their health. I will go into detail on this history later in the Enema section of this book. My personal and professional experience has shown me that colon cleansing can be a tremendously restorative tool in the face of our current lifestyle choices.

At the start of the OHC plan, a colon cleansing session is administered by a colon hydrotherapist or done by you using enemas. This internal cleansing provides the intestinal tract and the immune system with a "fresh start," since the water flushes out tremendous amounts of toxins, bacterial waste, and decaying particles residing in the colon. Most people feel physically refreshed after a colon cleansing session and are then motivated to start eating well for the first ten days to maintain that good feeling. Read the chapters on Colon Hydrotherapy and Therapeutic Enemas for further explanation.

Quick-Start Guide to the OHC Nutrition Program
The following quick-start guide will be explained in detail in the next chapter. Use this at-a-glance version as a reference guide.

FYI: Small farms are driven out of business and food variety decreases because it is dictated by shelf life. The "food fight" addresses not only what we eat in our homes, but also what our children eat in school. The natural foods movement includes farms, (some) colleges and universities, restaurants, retailers, and nonprofit organizations.

FYI: If you do not have access to colon hydrotherapy or you wish to spend your health dollars on organic foods, water filtration, raw dairy, or meat from grass-fed cattle, there is a chapter on enemas that will guide you in setting up your own in-home cleansing program that is equally as effective as having professional colon hydrotherapy.

As I have stated, the following program is based on the research of Dr. Price, as well as on many years of dedicated practice by alternative health practitioners. I know that this program will assist you in attaining your goals; I apply its principles at the OHC with new clients every week. It works. Foods do assist our bodies to heal.

Make a copy of the following Ten Day Nutritional Program to put on your refrigerator or somewhere you will be able to glance at it often. Alternatively, you can go to my Web site, where you can print it: www.optimalhealthnetwork.com/tendaydiet.htm.

Colon Hyrdrotherapy or Enemas?

Chapter Seven is devoted to colon hydrotherapy, and Chapter Eight covers therapeutic enemas. These colon cleanses are explained in detail so that readers will understand the differences between them. This is a self-help program that can be accomplished with at-home enemas, but it is also possible for a colon hydrotherapist to assist with the colon cleanses.

In addition to the details presented in this book, self-help instructional videos are available at my office, including:

All About Enemas Instructional Video or DVD
Cleansing, Coffee Enemas and Colon Tubes (Video)
Complete Colon Health 2-DVD Set

---

1. Water

   Drink "reverse osmosis" water all day long. Ideally, drink ½ cup every ½ hour, except at meals. For those of you who are drinking raw milk, you may replace some of the water with ½ to 2 cups of milk.

2. Breakfast

Eat breakfast every day. It is important that it consist of protein and fat.

3. Fruit

If you eat fruit during a day, only eat it 5-10 minutes before a meal.

4. Small Meals

Eat a small meal every 3-4 hours. This means that you will be eating 4-6 meals a day.

5. Non-Starchy Vegetables

Eat non-starchy vegetables 2-4 times daily. Organic (pesticide-free) is best. Eat greens every day. Non-starchy vegetables include: raw sauerkraut, broccoli, celery, peppers, tomatoes, zucchini, onions, spinach, salad greens, kale, spaghetti squash, cauliflower, bok choy, collard greens, and more.

6. Protein

Eat 5-25 grams of protein every 3-4 hours. Proteins may include: non-commercial, grass-fed meat such as beef or buffalo, ostrich, elk, raw dairy products, safe fish, organic chicken, organic turkey, and pasture-raised eggs. It is essential that you eat some animal protein and that you eat fat with your protein.

7. Healthy Fats

Eat healthy fats throughout the day. Healthy fats include, but are not limited to: grass-fed butter, grass-fed butter oil, grass-fed meat, ocean-caught fish, fish oils, cod liver oil, coconut oil, grass-fed ghee, avocados, flax-seed oil, pasture-raised eggs, olive oil, nuts, and seeds. Eat nuts and seeds, including flax seeds, in small amounts only.

FYI: Overcoming the potential hazards in genetically modified food, fish that is poisoned by mercury (or over-fished), and the hormones that have been added to dairy products is no small task. Besides risking your health, you may also be unwittingly injuring your local economy. For example, more and more cheap food is imported from countries outside the U.S. where labor is very cheap. This practice jeopardizes small family farms in favor of large corporate agriculture that pollutes our environment and contaminates the food chain with genetically engineered crops. When you purchase locally grown food, you save money by eliminating the companies in the middle of the distribution chain.

FYI: To avoid genetically modified food, print a copy of the True Food Network's non-genetically engineered (non-GE) brands and take it with you to the store. www.truefoodnow.com/shoppersguide.

8. Food With High Enzyme Content

Eat foods that have a high enzyme content: raw dairy, raw or lightly cooked non-commercial meats, and lacto-fermented food and drinks such as yogurt, kefir, raw cultured vegetables, and kvass.

9. Soups Made With Bone Broth

Eat soup that has been prepared using soup bones.

10. Raw Dairy

Eat raw dairy products.

Special Note on Detoxification

This OHC Plan has been carefully designed to support a healthy detoxification process without sending you into a state of illness. But it is also possible, given most people's diets and exposure to toxins, that a plan like this could trigger a health crisis. Even though you are eating food, this is a cleansing program. Because of this, and because we are all so toxic with yeast, PCBs, phenolics, heavy metals, and other toxins, it is very common to feel worse or even ill for the first 24 to 36 hours or even longer. In order to aid the liver in its enormous job of detoxifying your body, you may need to take coffee enemas as often as one to two times daily.

Shopping for Food

The two most important purposes of the OHC Ten-Day Plan are to rid the body of toxins and to deeply nourish the cells. During this time of cleansing and healing, your body will release many built-up toxins and increase its need for nutrients. By consuming only organic foods, you will reduce the intake of toxins and antibiotics into your system and take in more vitally needed vitamins, minerals, and phytonutrients. It is important that you do not eat anything that is counterproductive to the detoxifying and healing process. Organic foods are the best dietary choice for achieving the goals of this plan. Avoiding any contact with, or consumption of, chemicals and pesticides in our daily lives improves our chances for meeting our goals for optimal health.

You will find when you go shopping for the foods that you need to eat during this plan that commercial food is less expensive than organic food. However, commercial food can be very costly to your health in the long run, since it typically comes from sources that use a full spectrum of chemicals to control pests and bacteria and to increase production. Consuming the toxins used in those pesticides and herbicides, as well as the antibiotics used in meats, exposes your immune system and digestive tract to damaging toxins.

In addition to not ingesting harmful substances, you will reap a wealth of nutritional benefits from consuming only organic foods. Organic food has two to five times more nutrients than conventionally grown food. Because nutrients are the fuel of your cellular engines, maximizing nutrient intake gives you the best chance to reach your best possible health levels.

Healthy vs. Unhealthy Fats

Fats will be some of the most important products you purchase, and they are also the most confusing. As Sally Fallon's co-author, Dr. Mary Enig, explains, "As a result of being misled, we have a consuming public terrified of natural fats and oils—a public which, by its avoidance of these natural fats and oils, and consumption of fabricated, man-manipulated fat and oil replacements, such as the trans fats and the unstable polyunsaturates, is becoming increasingly obese and ill […] This attempt by the FDA to tar

FYI: Monterey Bay Aquarium's Seafood Watch Card, available on their Web site, contains directions for purchasing fish that's caught or farmed in ways that support healthy oceans. Go to www.mbay-aq.org/cr/seafoodwatch.asp to print out a copy of the card.

the wholesome saturated fats with the sins of the trans fats so as to promote in the minds of the consumers the idea that they are both the same, is not supported by real science. Biologically, the saturates and the trans have totally opposite effects; the effects of the saturates are good and those of the trans are undesirable."

1. Healthy Fats

High-quality animal fats are your best source of healthy fats.

Fats provide the essential nutrients for our cellular membranes, and our hormones and hormone-like substances. Fats are also our best tool for keeping our blood sugar balanced. High-quality animal fats are essential in the diet today. Raw, grass-fed, butter is our best health food. When heated, fats are altered thereby creating dangerous free radicals. In addition, when fats are heated, the life-giving elements of fats, like enzymes and the Wulzen factor, are destroyed. It is best not to heat fats. Healthy fats are high in essential nutrients needed to fight toxins and rebuild healthy, vibrant cells. Raw, organic, animal fats are your healthiest sources of fats. Other healthy fats include:

Avocado
Black Currant Oil
Borage Oil
Butter, grass-fed raw
Caviar
Coconut Oil
Cod Liver Oil
Egg Yolks, organic and raw
EPA Fish Oil
Evening Primrose Oil
Flax-Seed Oil
Fortified Flax
Ghee, raw
Grapeseed Oil
Nuts, soaked raw (not peanuts), very high in omega 6—
    use sparingly

Nut Butters, raw (not peanut butter), very high in omega-6,
   use sparingly
Olives, non-hybrid
Olive Oil, organic, expeller-pressed extra virgin
Raw or rare grass-fed buffalo or beef
Raw or rare ostrich or elk
Raw or rare fish
Seeds, soaked
Sesame Tahini

2. Acceptable Fats

This list includes fats that may have some toxic residue or
altered fat molecules, so they should be used more selectively.

Egg Yolks, commercial
Nut Butters, roasted
Olives
Peanut Oil
Pork Rinds
Safflower Oil (unrefined, expeller pressed)
Sesame Oil (unrefined, expeller pressed, limit use due to
   excess omega 6)
Spectrum Oil (by Spectrum Naturals)
Sunflower Oil (unrefined, expeller-pressed)

3. Unhealthy Fats

The following list of fats contains altered fat molecules that
lead to cellular damage. The damage occurs especially in the
organs and the immune/endocrine system.

Animal fats from animals raised on grains
Commercial Oil
Corn Oil
Cottonseed Oil
Deep fat frying oil (oil is overheated constantly, later "cleaned"
and reused again and again)
Fried Fats (overheated)

FYI: LocalHarvest.
org, founded in 1998 by
Guillermo Payet, a soft-
ware engineer and activ-
ist, is an online resource
for finding family farms
farmers markets, food
co-ops, and restaurants
that support local farm-
ers. LocalHarvest.com has
7,000 members and ten
new members are added
every day.

FYI: Farmer's markets are open-air street markets that provide farmers with a means to sell their produce directly to the public. According to the 2002 National Farmers Market Directory, there are over 3,100 farmers markets operating in the United States. Use the online database at www.localharvest.org to locate farmer's markets in your area.

Lard, commercial
Margarine (except for Spectrum Spread, a non-hydrogenated oil)
Oils, partially hydrogenated or hydrogenated
Shortening
Canola Oil
Oils that are chemically extracted or heated oils
Old oils
Soybean Oil

CHAPTER FOUR

Understanding the
Optimal Health Center (OHC)
Nutrition Program

"According to a USDA study on nutrition, major health issues are diet-related and the solution to illness can be found in nutrition. The real potential from improved diet is preventative in that it may defer or modify the development of a disease state. These findings are corroborated by Surgeon General C. Everett Koop's 1988 Report on Nutrition and Health."

- Mary Enig, Ph.D.,
Science Advisor and Vice President
Weston A. Price Foundation

FYI: Food cooperatives are membership-based buying organizations that distribute natural food products to consumers. Most co-ops were founded during the 1960s and 1970s to offer natural foods that most supermarkets would not sell. Co-ops are community-run, community-controlled enterprises. There are approximately 500 retail cooperative food stores in the United States committed to consumer education, service, product quality, truth in advertising, and member control. Co-ops are open to non-members, but the benefits of membership include a vote, discounts, and other services.

Chapter Four included a Quick Start Guide to the OHC nutrition guidelines that will be described in detail in this chapter. Although the guidelines are designed for a 35-day cleansing and nutrition program, many people find that they want to integrate the principles into their lifestyle permanently. When you get past the release of toxins in the first week, there's a surge of energy and alertness and a sense of well-being that motivates you more than anything that you read or hear.

Adopting a New Normal

The transition to healthy eating involves a change in food buying patterns and more cooking. In some ways, the 35-day OHC cleansing and nutrition plan challenges you to make changes that are immediate, and a healthy body motivates you to keep going. If you fall back into previous unhealthy eating habits, you'll be able to notice a difference in how you feel. In a way, bad eating habits

FYI: Although many large supermarkets have added organic foods to their shelves, the selection is often limited. Large chain stores ought to be the last place you shop. Here's why:

Concentration on Retailing Destroys Communities
Large chains do not source locally because they need suppliers who can supply identical products to all their stores.

Large Chains Destroy Small Businesses
Retail profits do not go to a local area but to shareholders who have no interest in local communities. By contrast, the money you spend locally circulates dollars in your community and generates jobs.

Multinational Trade Means Greater Food Transport
Supermarkets prefer to do business with major players—even if they are around the globe. This means that the food will be transported long distances, contributing to excessive use of fuel and resultant global warming.

will be self-correcting if you prefer health over the yucky feeling that occurs when you eat the wrong foods.

Water

Essential Guideline:
Drink "reverse osmosis" or spring water all day. Three quarts or roughly ½ cup every ½ an hour. Raw milk can be substituted for some water.

Additional Details:

- Drinking enough of the right kind of water is essential to optimal health. Water is the medium in which all metabolic actions take place. Every cell depends upon water for carrying out its life-giving functions; our kidneys, liver, lungs, and skin rely upon these metabolic processes to do their job of clearing the body of waste and toxins. By consuming water on a regular basis, such as the recommended ½ cup of water every half hour, you will help your body keep toxins out of your cells, as well as removing currently stored toxins. If you find drinking nothing but water a little boring during the day, treat yourself to a cup of herbal tea, but make sure that at least 2-3 quarts of the water you drink consists of quality, plain water. (The general rule for adequate water consumption is one quart of quality water per 50 pounds of body weight.)

- Well-water may be drunk for good health. However, make sure that you have your well-water tested for nitrates, nitrites, lead, and pesticides. There are many inexpensive tests on the market. People who live in the country and have clean water have highly beneficial minerals in their water. This water is healthier than filtered water.

- You want to steer clear of tap water because it contains chlorine and may contain fluoride and other toxic substances that, with ongoing consumption, can have grim consequences for the body. Distilled water should also be avoided because it has the wrong ionization, pH, and polarization and oxidation potentials, and can deplete your body of necessary minerals. Furthermore, distilled water has been tied to hair loss, which is often associated with mineral deficiencies.

- Reverse Osmosis is the most effective method of water filtration. It filters water by squeezing water through a semi-permeable membrane, which is rated at 0.0001 micron (equal to 0.00000004 inch!). This is the technology used to make bottled water, and it is also the only technology capable of desalinating sea water, which turns it into drinking water.

- Non-reverse osmosis water filters are much less effective, and the pore size on these filter media are much bigger, generally 0.5 - 10 micron. They can filter out coarse particles, sediments, and elements only up to their micron rating. Anything finer than this, and most dissolved substances cannot be filtered out. As a result, water filtered this way is far less clean and safe compared to reverse osmosis filtration.

- Spring water should be bottled in clear polyethylene or glass containers, not the one-gallon plastic (PVC) containers that transmit far too many chemicals into the water.

- For some, drinking water often can be the most daunting of all the tasks of this program, but keep in mind that this program is designed to set up new habits for your entire life. Don't fret. Develop an attitude of gracious persistence towards yourself: know you will succeed and know that it may take you a bit of time. Carry a water bottle with you at all times. I recommend drinking room-temperature water because ice-cold water can damage the delicate lining of your stomach.

- Be particular about the size of your water bottle. If it is hard for you to keep track of how much water you are drinking, make sure that the water bottle is a larger one that you need to refill only once or twice. Set your watch timer to go off every half-hour. And always remember, these guidelines are charming places to head towards, not prisons!

FYI: The Cooperative Grocer is a bimonthly magazine produced for the managers and directors of food cooperatives across the United States and Canada. The Cooperative Grocer Web site contains an online database that you can use to search for a food co-op in your area: www.cooperativegrocer.coop/coops.

Breakfast

Essential Guideline:
Eat breakfast within a half-hour of waking. Eating breakfast is a key part of the OHC plan! Your breakfast should consist of ¼ to one whole piece of fruit, followed 5-10 minutes later by non-

FYI: *Your Body's Many Cries for Water* by Dr. F. Batmanghelidj, MD, is devoted to the critical importance of water. See www.watercure.com.

starchy vegetables, fat, and protein. Not eating breakfast is a major factor in jeopardizing health.

Additional Details:

- Upon waking, your body needs nutrients. During a good night's sleep, your body has used up a rich supply of nutrients, helping it recover from the work of the previous day. Also, it has used nutrients to heal and rejuvenate stressed or damaged body parts. If you don't take steps to replenish those expended nutrients, the body will resort to utilizing its reserved store of nutrients. You don't want your body to have to run your day-to-day activities on those reserves. You want those reserves for times of crisis. You want those reserves for your own protection when others around you are sick, and of course, for graceful aging.

- A useful analogy that we are all familiar with regarding our body depleting its reserves is osteoporosis. Calcium, an essential mineral for many bodily functions, is stolen from the bones when the body becomes too acidic. An acidic body is caused by many factors, including not eating breakfast, staying up too late, and eating processed sugar and flour. When the body doesn't have the resources to counteract stressors, it steals from within itself to bring about homeostasis. Unfortunately, this imbalance often doesn't show up for many years, until one actually has osteoporosis.

- One of the most important things you can do for your health is to think about what you are eating and how it affects the balance of your blood sugar. Without breakfast, you start the day in a state of low blood sugar. Low blood sugar is always hard on the body. It can cause premature aging and adrenal exhaustion, and it pushes people towards binge eating of high-carbohydrate foods. Binge eating of carbohydrates sends a person's blood sugar into the too-high range. The subsequent effect is equivalent to riding a roller coaster all day long. The discipline of eating breakfast helps you eat better the rest of the day. When we take eating seriously, we ingest a higher quality, and more appropriate quantity, of necessary nutrients.

Fruit

Essential Guideline:
If you eat fruit at all, eat fruit five to ten minutes before meals only. Not everyone needs fruit.

Additional Details:

- Eating fruit before a meal can "kick start" your digestive process, encouraging better digestion of the food you eat afterwards. When you eat fruit five to ten minutes before a meal, the body is assisted with critical digestive energy in the form of fructose and enzymes. This prepares your body to use these by-products to break down food and extract nutrients from your carbohydrates, fats and protein, with less wasted energy and intestinal stress.

- Fruit digests more quickly than most other foods. When you eat fruit after a meal or as part of a dish, it sits in your stomach too long, where it putrefies and has a negative impact on your health. In addition, if you eat fruit alone, with no other food, it throws your blood sugar levels out of balance.

- Fruit juices should not be consumed because fruit juices do not have the fiber of the fruit. When you drink the juice without the fiber, large amounts of sugar flow into your blood stream too quickly. Your blood sugar rises, which is counterproductive; in order to be healthy, you need to always keep your blood sugar in balance.

- Fruit juices have too many carbohydrates. A re-balancing program such as the OHC Plan keeps the carbohydrate intake at a low level. In this way, your intestinal tract has a chance to re-balance its ecosystem with healthy microbes and to diminish the number of unhealthy microbes.

- For most participants starting the first ten-day period of the Optimal Health Center Plan, consuming 10 grams of carbohydrates in fruit at the beginning of a meal, six times a day, is ideal. Some individuals may need to adjust this intake amount based on their specific needs and any changes that occur during the program. For instance, a person with blood sugar imbal-

FYI: A key ingredient to the success of the OHC plan is to always know where your next meal is coming from. Finding yourself hungry, and not knowing what you are going to eat, is a recipe for giving up on this plan. When you cook, prepare large amounts of food. This will give you leftovers. Breakfast is a great time to eat the leftover stir fry or soup from last night's dinner. Also, you may need to bring food with you when you go out. Although, many restaurants serve excellent vegetable and protein dishes, skip the bread, potatoes, rice, pasta, and dessert.

FYI: Vitamin B12 that is available in meat, eggs and milk is used to produce the myelin sheath. Adequate levels of B12 can improve cognitive function.

ances may eat only 5 grams of carbohydrates in fruits, whereas an athlete may eat as many as 20 grams.

- During this plan, please stay away from dried fruit and melons. These foods often contain molds that can be harmful to your health. The other fruits to limit are bananas, mangoes, and other high-carbohydrate fruits. Look at the following comparison of the carbohydrate content of apples and bananas to see which fruit to consume. For example, a medium-size apple has about 15 grams of carbohydrates, while a medium-size banana, at 40 grams of carbohydrates, has two to three times the amount of needed fruit carbohydrates for one meal. If you choose to eat a banana, one-quarter to one-half a banana is a healthier selection.

Small Meals

Essential Guideline:
Eat a small meal every three to four hours. You will be eating four to six meals a day.

Additional Details:

- Since smaller quantities of consumed food are apt to flow through the digestive system without becoming toxic, it makes sense that we eat food in proportions that improve our digestive abilities rather than put a strain them.

- Providing the body with a continuous supply of usable nutrients throughout the day allows individual body systems to function with efficiency. This way your blood sugar level will remain more consistent and spare your body from the typical unhealthy fluctuations you have been subjecting it to for years. A second key reason for eating every few hours is to keep the adrenal glands in top shape. When you eat infrequently, you force your body to run on adrenaline.

- Modern living easily drains our adrenal glands. The adrenal glands, located one on top of each kidney, are stress glands that help us cope with internal and external stress factors, both physical and mental. Additional jobs of the adrenal glands include:

a) Manufacturing mineral corticoids, which balance all the minerals (builders and communicators) in the body. For instance, mineral corticoids help insure calcium is absorbed into the bones and magnesium to the muscles. Mineral corticoids balance our electrical system with sodium and potassium so that our nerve impulses are adequate. Mineral corticoids manage our salt and water balance to prevent water retention.

b) Producing glucocorticoids, which help our pancreas and liver coordinate insulin production with glucose levels in our blood. They help prevent overproduction of insulin, which can exhaust the pancreas and, in turn, the individual. The adrenal glands must be functioning well for us to have optimal amounts of energy.

c) Making cortisol, which is our natural antipain, anti-inflammatory, anti-allergy, and mood-elevation hormone.

d) Producing sexual steroidal hormones, which communicate to the male and female organs to promote healthy functioning. For example, in women, after menopause, adrenals should produce adequate levels of estrogen, and in men, they keep male hair growth patterns youthful.

• Given the stress inherent in modern living, it is essential to give the body adequate nutrition to lessen chances of adrenal exhaustion; and, in many cases, to assist the healing of the adrenal glands themselves. Persistent fatigue, a racing brain, an inability to "turn off" the feeling of being stressed out, as well as a lack of vitality, all point to adrenal exhaustion. The good news is that by keeping your blood sugar balanced, by eating small amounts of food often, and by eating animal protein throughout the day, you can keep your adrenal glands in a vital state of health.

FYI: Kombucha is a fermented health drink made from tea, sugar, and a culture called a *scoby*. Although there is no fruit in kombucha, it has a fizzy apple-cider taste. It is thought to have originated in the Far East, where it has been consumed for at least two thousand years. The first recorded use of kombucha comes from China in 221 B.C. during the Tsin Dynasty.

- Abuse of the adrenal glands can cause disease and a lack of healing in almost any part of the body. Even though adrenal exhaustion often presents itself with specific symptoms in some people, it will often be a less clearly defined aspect of many other diseases. For instance, research has shown:

  "...a significant association between variation of salivary cortisol throughout the day in patients with metastatic breast cancer and their subsequent survival." In short, the health of the adrenal glands determines overall health and overall ability to heal from many diseases.

  - Journal of the National Cancer Institute June 21, 2000;92:994-1000

- Recognizing that we are all unique in our food needs, the actual size, as well as the ratio of macronutrients, (carbohydrates to proteins to fats), of meals consumed every three to four hours can vary.

- Eat what will keep you satisfied for three to four hours. If after a meal you have an adverse symptom or worsening of existing negative symptoms, including: specifically sweet cravings, hunger too soon after eating, lowered energy, worsening moods, and others, then you are not eating the correct foods in appropriate ratios at your meal.

- If toward the end of your meal, you find yourself full and yet you continue to eat until you are stuffed, then you are not eating the right proportions of macronutrients. My general principle here is to start by cutting down on your carbohydrates. Also, keep in mind that the meal size and proportions can change throughout the plan as your body accommodates the cumulative effects of the entire OHC Plan. Feel free to call or e-mail if you need further assistance. I would be honored to work with you one-on-one.

- Again, given how much stress is inherent in modern living, "having" to eat every few hours can appear impossible. But it is important to remember that you are at an exciting point in your life where you are changing habits, and that this takes time. Generally speaking, as people incorporate these lifestyle changes into their day-to-day lives, they will be challenged emotionally.

- As you proceed, you may find that you have largely chosen what to eat based on your feelings, not on what foods would bring you optimal health. As you make this plan your way of life, your feelings will come to the fore. Feelings are healthy. Feelings are normal. Use them as guides to deeper healing. Talk to friends. Cry a lot. Laugh deeply. Rage into your pillow. And be deeply kind to yourself. You're asking a lot of yourself.

Non-Starchy Vegetables

Essential Guideline:

Eat non-starchy vegetables two to four times daily. Eating vegetables throughout the day will optimize your bodily systems and functions.

Additional Details:

- Green and non-starchy vegetables contain vitamins, minerals, phytonutrients, chlorophyll, fibers, and carbohydrates that your body needs to function efficiently and keep its systems in balance. The nutrients in vegetables activate the energies in the body necessary for cleansing and rebuilding. At least two of your meals should consist of non-starchy vegetables. For some, as many as four to five servings of non-starchy vegetables a day is optimal.

- Vegetables are important for many reasons and one of these is that they are loaded with fiber. The fiber acts as a biochemical sponge for the body, absorbing impurities, gases, and toxins. It also decreases the amount of time in which the stool is in contact with the colon wall, thereby minimizing the colon's exposure to carcinogens. Finally, fiber fills our bodies up without raising the blood sugar level.

- Recommended non-starchy vegetables include but are not limited to: broccoli, cucumbers, celery, peppers, tomatoes, spinach, green beans, peas, zucchini, onions, salad greens, dandelion

FYI: Kefir is a family of fermented beverages made from kefir grains including a yogurt-like drink with a slightly fizzy taste and a water-kefir that has no dairy content. Kefir's history dates back several centuries. Its origin is thought to be the Caucasus mountains in Central Asia, where tribespeople drink kefir instead of water and eat thickened kefir in place of a dessert. Their life expectancy is between 110 and 150 years.

Try to be asleep by 10 p.m. Critical repair of the entire body, and specifically of the adrenal glands, occurs from 11 p.m. to 1 a.m. If you are awake, this healing does not occur. In addition, your gallbladder dumps toxins from 11 p.m. to 1 a.m. If you are awake, the toxins back up into the liver, which then back up into your system and cause further disruption of your health. While cleansing, it is imperative that the toxins you are releasing from your cells are not being recirculated throughout your body. You might even consider starting this sleep program a month before you start your cleanse so that your body will be strong enough to do the work of the cleanse.

greens, kale, spaghetti squash, cauliflower, bok choy, and collard greens. For many people, it will be best to eat some of the vegetables raw (as with all other food on this diet) whenever possible.

- Remember that eating some foods raw is one of the principles of traditional cultures. In the event that your digestive system is unable to handle raw vegetables, you may need to steam or cook your vegetables, although cooking has a tendency to leach many of the valuable nutrients from the vegetables. This is okay, as long as you are eating some of your foods raw, like your dairy goods, fruits, avocados, meats, and fermented foods.

- The vegetable juicer and the Vita Mix are both great options to consider when increasing your vegetable consumption. If you have access to a juicer or a juice bar, you may find that you will absolutely thrive by drinking at least 16 ounces of mostly non-starchy vegetable juice daily. The Vita Mix is like a blender, but if turns large amounts of vegetables into a creamy raw soup. These tools will easily increase your vegetable consumption.

Protein

Essential Guideline:
Eat a handful-size portion of protein (5-25 grams), every three to four hours.

Additional Details:

- The most fundamental building block of the traditional diet was animal products. No traditional culture has ever nourished itself exclusively on plant foods.

- Although the proportion of animal protein to other foods in the diet varied considerably, the diet of some Eskimo groups has consisted of almost 100 percent animal products. African tribes ate entire animals, including raw liver. Natives of the Polynesian islands ate lots of seafood. Other tribes ate raw grubs and insects.

- Use your body's cellular need for protein as a guide. How much protein is ideal for each person is confusing, but it need not be. When we look at how much protein is eaten in the United States, it would seem that most of us are getting enough, but it is the individual cellular need for protein that is at issue, and not the volume of protein consumed.

FYI: Dr. Joseph Mercola is an osteopath in Chicago who has built one of the largest alternative health Web sites on the Internet: www.mercola.com. I highly recommend his bi-weekly newsletter.

- Most people are actually protein-deficient at the cellular level. Experts who say people get too much protein are basing this evaluation on the products of protein elimination. What the experts ought to be saying is that people assimilate too little of the protein they eat, with the result that most consumed protein turns toxic and over-stresses our elimination systems.

- If we look to scientific research to determine if people are getting enough protein, what do we find? The following quote will help you to understand why it is not common knowledge that you need more protein, or amino acids, than you may be eating:

"The requirements for the indispensable amino acids have been determined by a number of different methods. Historically, descriptive or gross measures like growth and nitrogen balance have been used. However, technological advancements in recent years have resulted in the use of more precise and mechanistic metabolic approaches (i.e., plasma amino acid concentrations, amino acid oxidation, indicator amino acid oxidation) to examine requirements. Nevertheless, the current recommendations are still based on nitrogen balance studies. Requirement estimates based on other methodologies, such as plasma amino acid concentrations and direct amino acid oxidation, suggest that the requirement estimates derived from nitrogen balance experiments are too low."

- American Journal of Clinical Nutrition, Vol. 74, No. 6, 756-760, December 2001.

- For certain, most healers know that it is critical for those who are in a state of rebuilding, repairing and cleansing to get ample amounts of the right kinds of protein.

- Protein deficiencies contribute to mood disorders, digestion problems, hormonal imbalances, cardiovascular problems, detoxification problems, pH imbalances, and muscular-skeletal disorders. In addition, insulin intolerance, a pre-diabetic condition, is an important factor influencing your body's need for amino acids. Also, it is important to know that if you eat sugar, you will need more protein than if you don't eat sugar. Just this fact alone points to a higher need for quality protein for most people today.

- When a person is sick and/or on a cleansing and rebuilding regime, such as the OHC plan, the proper levels of protein are essential because amino acids help in the exchange of nutrients and wastes between cells and the intercellular fluids.

- Even scientific research shows us that "the dietary 'essentiality' of a given amino acid is dependent on the ratio of supply to demand (in the individual body); the distinction between 'essential' and 'nonessential' largely disappears because it is dependent on conditions." Since most people have spent years eating lower-quality proteins and a diet based on carbohydrates, it is essential to your long-term health that you nourish yourself with high-quality proteins in order to rebuild your health and cleanse your system.

- Amino acids are "building blocks of proteins" and combine in thousands of ways in order to produce all of our enzymes, hormones, and neurotransmitters, as well as to build every structural part of our bodies, including the skeletal structure of our cells (*Biochemistry*, Second Edition, Matthews, Van Holde, 1996). Thus, protein could appropriately be considered "the most valuable player" for every bodily system or function. Even though most of the amino acids can be manufactured by the body itself, there are eight amino acids that the body can't produce and that therefore must be obtained from the protein that we eat. These eight are called the *essential amino acids*.

- Only animal protein possesses the eight essential amino acids in the quantities and proportions necessary to accomplish the healing process. If we don't take in the amino acids that our bodies need and can easily use, our detoxification systems cannot fully function.

- Though some people argue that one can get the essential amino acids by combining various plant sources of protein, dependence on plant sources alone for essential amino acids is problematic for a number of reasons:

  1) Many plant sources of protein contain such small quantities of protein in comparison to their carbohydrate content, that one would have to ingest an excessive amount of carbohydrate foods just to ingest enough essential amino acids.

  2) Many people are not able to digest protein very well. Depending on only plant sources of protein to get therapeutic amounts of certain amino acids often overloads your system with toxic nutrients. For example, if you rely on nuts and seeds as a primary protein source, you are altering your body's ratio of omega 3 to omega 6 fats, creating an imbalance. This imbalance of omega 3 to omega 6 fatty acids is now known to cause many health problems.

  3) Due to the amount of stress most of us are under in the modern world, our livers are being excessively taxed. The amino acids, l-methionine, l-glutathione, and l-glutamine, all of which are found in abundance in animal protein, need to be consumed in therapeutic amounts. Without animal protein in your diet, it is very difficult to do this.

- Many people who prefer to eat plant protein eat a lot of soy and they don't realize it is deficient in the sulfur-containing amino acids, methionine and cysteine. In the United States, soy foods are highly processed, which denatures the protein and increases levels of carcinogens. In addition, soy contains lots of phytoestrogens that have negative hormonal effects, as well as trypsin inhibitors that inhibit protein digestion and affect pancreatic function. Soy foods can also cause deficiencies in calcium and vitamin D. People with thyroid problems need to avoid soy altogether. Finally, it is now thought that soy foods consumed in large amounts may contribute to cancer.

- Those who eat soy often point to its consumption in Asia. Although it is true that soy is part of the Asian diet, tradition-

FYI: Kefir's live yeast and bacteria cultures can colonize the intestinal tract to control and eliminate destructive pathogenic microorganisms. When this happens, the body becomes more efficient in resisting such pathogens as E. coli and intestinal parasites.

ally it was eaten in its fermented state, processed to remove the toxins, and eaten with meat. In Japan it is eaten with fish, and in China, with pork. It is not considered a replacement for animal foods and never constitutes more than 1 to 2% of total caloric intake. In Japan, the average consumption of soy is 10 grams—about two teaspoons—per day. The same is true of China. In short, although Asians include soy in their diet, they consider it a condiment and eat it in small amounts—never as a staple.

• When I endorse animal products, I explain the extreme importance of seeking out the highest-quality foods, sometimes going to great lengths to do so. Typically, in the United States what we mean by eating protein is the consumption of lots of grain-fed, antibiotic- and hormone-laden, and over-processed beef, pork, chicken, and dairy products. In addition to being pumped full of unhealthy substances, cows, pigs and chickens are most often left in cages, without any access to their traditional diets or sunshine.

• Poor-quality meats contain antimicrobial drugs that were given to the animals when they were raised. Because we don't raise meat animals in accordance to inherent health needs, we are forced to keep them alive by using the anti-microbials. The horror of this situation is that we are making the very pathogens that we are trying to control even more deadly. The continued use of these anti-microbial drugs on the animal products we eat is forcing the known pathogens to mutate into newer strains that are resistant to existing drugs. We are actually creating a future health nightmare via commercial meats. This process is paving the way for new strains of deadly pathogens, which current medicine has no antibiotics to fight. Research from the FDA backs this up:

"The consumption of animal products contaminated with bacteria may compromise human health. Changes in animals' enteric bacteria, including pathogen load and development of anti-microbial resistance, may occur as a result of anti-microbial use in food producing animals."

– FDA Guidance for Industry #78

- According to the renowned cancer specialist, Virginia Livingston-Wheeler:

    "…most chicken and nearly half the beef consumed in America today is cancerous and pathogenic. Her research has convinced her that these cancers are transmissible to man."

    -Nourishing Traditions, Sally Fallon

- As we all know, our oceans have been contaminated with many toxins, such as mercury, that can be extremely detrimental to our health.

- When I recommend animal protein, I mean safe fish, organic, pasture-raised eggs, pasture-raised or grass-fed, non-grain-fed, lamb, ostrich, elk, buffalo, beef, goat, chicken, turkey, and wild game. This list would also include dairy from pasture fed cows, goats and sheep.

- The key to acquiring healthy meat is to seek out grass-fed animal products from a local farmer who is raising the animals, and to develop a relationship with him or her to make sure that you can confirm how the animals are raised. In such a situation, you don't have to be concerned about government organic certification, but rather have the farmer let you know about the organic status of their individual farm. Unfortunately, most natural food stores don't sell grass-fed meats. Their beef is only marginally better than commercial meats. Don't pay twice as much for your meat and continue to get inferior quality.

- Pasture-fed animals eliminate all possibility of cows carrying Mad Cow Disease because the cattle eat only grasses, hay, and grass silage. Mad Cow Disease, or bovine spongiform encephalopathy, BSE, is thought to come from cattle being fed meat and bone meal made from other cattle that have been infected with BSE. In addition, pasture-fed animals have far fewer E. coli than grain-fed animals. An overgrowth of E. coli in cattle is similar to yeast overgrowth in humans. If you feed cows what they are supposed to eat grass—their inner ecology is not overrun with unhealthy organisms.

FYI: Today five giant farms control fully one-half of the $400 million organic produce market in California. Partly as a result, the price premium for organic crops is shrinking. This is all to the good for expanding organic's market beyond yuppies, but it is crushing many of the small farmers for whom organic has represented a profitable niche, a way out of the cheap-food economics that has ravaged American farming over the last few decades.

Michael Pollan
"Behind the Organic-Industrial Complex"

- Again, it is important to know the fact that not one plan fits all when it comes to protein consumption. Protein needs vary according to one's age and activity. For some participants, just eating an organic egg or two, a cup of raw cream, a full glass of raw milk, and some chicken broth throughout the day, supplemented with nuts and seeds, is plenty of animal protein. Another person may find he needs as much as 2 servings of lamb, 4 oz of fish, a few slices of raw cheese, a handful of pumpkin seeds and a serving of grass-fed beef all in the same day.

- You may need to take a Betaine and Pepsin supplement along with cayenne pepper or lemon juice to optimize your ability to digest protein. Or, you may need to eat your non-commercial meats raw or rare.

- Raw meats were eaten by all cultures studied by Dr. Price. For that matter, most cultures throughout the world still have some raw meat in their dietary fare; sushi, carpaccio, kebbeh, and steak tartare are a few examples.

- Raw meat rebuilds and repairs the body better than any other food. I, personally, was not able to heal, even after working diligently on my health for over six years, until I ate large quantities of raw meat.

- Raw meat has traditionally been humankind's main source of the heat-sensitive pyridoxine, or B6, in addition to healing fats. (I will go into the healing value of fats in the next section.) Unfortunately, raw liver, which has historically been our richest source of B6, is no longer widely consumed.

- The astronomical prevalence of yeast overgrowth is one health issue that can be directly linked to B6 deficiency. In addition:

    "...deficiencies of B6 have been linked with diabetes, heart disease, nervous disorders, carpel tunnel syndrome, PMS, morning sickness, toxemia of pregnancy, kidney failure, alcoholism, sickle cell anemia, and cancer."

    - Nourishing Traditions, by Sally Fallon
    Raw Meat Appetizers section

- Eating raw meat or at least rare meats, including organ meats, will dramatically improve your health. When you have food cravings, are tired, weak, or when your concentration is poor, reach for protein. Protein helps keep that all-important blood sugar in balance. Eating protein at every meal is required for optimal health. Eat animal protein for at least one, if not all, of your meals. Doing this prevents deficiency of protein, as well as giving the detoxification system the therapeutic level of nutrients that it needs.

- It is possible to be a healthy vegetarian and follow this plan, but you will need to consume the right quantities of both protein and fat from raw, grass-fed butter, cream and milk, and pasture-raised raw eggs. However, some of you will need to take in as much as a ½ a pound or more of butter daily and 10-20 eggs per week. And these eggs do need to be raw and pasture-raised. In addition, it is best if they have been fertilized by a rooster and never refrigerated. Make sure that the egg yolk is bright orange and that the white has two distinctive sections. And, of course, whether or not you can be optimally healthy and a vegetarian is determined by your own body.

"In order to utilize these minerals, and to build and maintain the functions of various organs, definite quantities of various organic catalysts which act as activating substances are needed."

> - Weston A Price
> Nutrition and Physical
> Degeneration

FYI: In Maine, Eliot Coleman has pioneered a sophisticated market garden entirely under plastic, to supply his "food shed" with local produce all winter long; even in January his solar-heated farm beats California on freshness and quality, if not price.

Michael Pollan
"Behind the Organic-Industrial Complex"

Healthy Fats and Oil

Essential Guideline:
Eat Healthy Fat and Oil throughout the Day. Fats and oils are our most important nutrient.

Additional Details:

- You cannot be healthy without significant amounts of high-quality, raw fats and oils in your daily diet, fats are required by our bodies to cleanse, to repair, and to rebuild.

- Today, people are more deficient in fat and oil than in any other nutrient. If we think logically, we know this. We live in a fat-phobic world where fat is one of only three macronutrients: carbohydrates, protein, and fats. We need all of these three macronutrients.

- Unfortunately, the importance of fats and oils in the human diet has only become widely recognized within the last few years; most people have been erroneously convinced that fats and oils are damaging to one's health. This is a lie. Why is sufficient fat and oil consumption necessary to be optimally healthy and/or for a complete restoration of health?

- It is important to eat a large amount of your healthy fats and oils raw. Raw fats are crucial for health because they contain lipase, the fat-splitting enzyme. Lipase prepares the fat you eat so that it may be utilized by the cells and the organs. Without sufficient lipase in your body, your body cannot properly utilize the fats that you eat and your pancreas becomes over-worked.

- Healthy fats and oils replenish our cellular membranes with needed nutrients. It is the fats that keep our cell walls strong. By maintaining the structural integrity of our cells, fats promote the full functioning of our rebuilding and cleansing mechanisms. The cell's ability to renew itself keeps us young and healthy.

- The diets of healthy native groups contained at least ten times more vitamin A and vitamin D than the American diet during the 1930's (Pay attention here! The people in the 1930s didn't live in a fat-phobic culture. Everyone was drinking whole milk and eating butter at every meal!) Vitamins A and D are found only in animal fats—butter, lard, egg yolks, fish oils, and foods with fat-rich cellular membranes like liver, and other organ meats, fish eggs, and shell fish.

- Fats and oils are our only source of the omega-3 essential fatty acid. It has been estimated that less than 30 percent of Americans consume an adequate supply of omega-3 fatty acids. Omega-3s are essential fatty acids due to the vital role they play in every cell and system in your body. People who have ample amounts of omega-3s in their diet are less likely to have high blood pressure and are 50 percent less likely to suffer a heart attack. Essential fatty acids also attract oxygen and aid in its transport to needed organs and even to individual cells throughout the body. Oxygenation is crucial for obtaining a state of optimal health.

FYI: High cholesterol is not the cause of heart disease. In spite of the official advice that tells us to lower the amount of saturated fat in our diet, we have an epidemic amount of heart disease.

- Toxins, in order to leave our bodies, need to be taken from the cells and bound to a carrier of toxins. Most cleansing programs only carry toxins out of the main circulation. How do we get toxins out of the places where they are stored? Eat high-quality, raw fats. Fats are binding agents. Fats bind toxins more than any other substance.

- Many toxins are actually fat-seeking. Dioxin is one of these lipophilic toxins, meaning that it seeks fat. All of us have dioxin in our systems, along with hundreds of other toxic chemicals that are fat-seeking. Most of us don't and haven't ingested enough high-quality fat over the years to safely remove the toxins that are stored in our bodies. This is an absolutely essential reason to increase your fat and oil intake.

- Saturated fats from animal sources—portrayed as the enemy by the United States Food and Drug Administration and consequently by American culture—give the body the raw materials it demands from us in order to be optimally healthy. Saturated fats form an important part of the cellular membrane by giving the cellular membrane rigidity; they protect the immune system and enhance the utilization of essential fatty acids. Saturated fats are needed for the proper development of the brain and nervous systems.

- Certain types of saturated fats provide quick energy and protect against pathogenic microorganisms in the intestinal tract. Other types of saturated fat provide energy to the heart.

FYI: I've found that people who are chronically ill and who are not recovering their health even though they are following a rigorous program do heal when they take in more of the fat-soluble vitamins. You won't heal fully or stay vibrantly healthy if you don't absorb your food. You can't absorb your food without the proper amounts of vitamin A, vitamin D, and Activator X. It is possible that you may need to start with at least one stick of raw butter a day, along with copious amounts of cod liver oil, raw cream, avocados, and coconut oil.

- One saturated fat we are all familiar with is cholesterol. Cholesterol is the precursor to bile acids, which are needed to digest and absorb long-chain fatty acids. Cholesterol is also recognized for its physiological importance in the skin and the intestines where it plays an important structural role as a component of the organ membranes.

- Cells lining the digestive tract are particularly rich in cholesterol. Among its other various roles in the cell are the signaling activities that, for example, tell the gastrointestinal musculature when to contract. I don't know how many people I have seen relieved of their chronic constipation, as well as any related Irritable Bowel Syndrome (IBS), when they finally ate enough cholesterol in their daily diet.

- Cholesterol is responsible for our sex and adrenal hormones. It is also one of our primary repair mechanisms, which is why our arteries end up with patches of repairing cholesterol. Low-density lipoproteins, or LDL, carries cholesterol to the cells, which means that our LDL numbers need to be high enough.

- Our livers—and not our food—make the cholesterol that our body uses for repair.

- Foods high in cholesterol help to repair the liver. As the body heals, it needs more cholesterol to repair the liver and to replace broken-down cells.

- Even the Framingham studies, which the pharmaceutical companies use to promote cholesterol-lowering drugs, show that the higher the cholesterol level and the more fat in the diet, the longer the study participants lived and the more optimally the participants weighed.

- Fats are the macronutrient that allows us to feel full, to minimize food cravings, and to most fully meet the energy needs of our organs. Our bodies use fats as a supply and store of energy: a gram of fat contains more than double the amount of energy present in a gram of carbohydrate.

- Given that we live in a fat-phobic world, it is no wonder that so many people are struggling with such diseases as Chronic

Weston A. Price's Thoughts on Fat-Soluble Vitamins

Price referred to these fat-soluble vitamins as "catalysts," or "activators" upon which the assimilation of all the other nutrients depended—protein, minerals, and water-soluble vitamins. In other words, without sufficient quantities of vitamins A and D in the diet, the body is significantly challenged to utilize the water-soluble vitamins, proteins, and minerals.

"There are a number of factors that can prevent the uptake of minerals, even when they are available in our food. The glandular system that regulates the messages sent to the intestinal mucosa requires plentiful fat-soluble vitamins in the diet to work properly. Likewise, the intestinal mucosa requires fat-soluble vitamins and adequate dietary cholesterol to maintain proper integrity so that it passes only those nutrients the body needs, while at the same time keeping out toxins and large, undigested proteins that can cause allergic reactions."

> *- Nourishing Traditions by Sally Fallon and Mary G. Enig, PhD. www.westonaprice. org/nutrition guidelines/mineralprimer.html*

Price also discovered another fat-soluble vitamin that was a more powerful catalyst for nutrient absorption than vitamins A and D. He called it "Activator X." All the healthy groups Price studied had the Activator X in their diets. It is found in certain special foods that these people considered Sacred—cod liver oil, fish eggs, organ meats, and the deep-yellow Spring and Fall butter from cows eating rapidly growing green grass.

FYI: The movie we have produced called, *Cleansing, Coffee Enemas and Colon Tubes*, teaches how to remove toxins from your body. Look for it at www.optimalhealth-network.com

Fatigue Syndrome and with such physical challenges such as feeling constantly hungry, even after they have eaten.

- Our organs are made up of lots of fats; your liver is made of 80% fat. You must eat raw fat in order to regenerate your organs, including the liver.

- Prostaglandins are a group of about a dozen compounds synthesized from fatty acids. Prostaglandins are highly potent substances that are not stored but are produced as needed by cell membranes in virtually every body tissue. Different prostaglandins have been found to raise or lower blood pressure, regulate smooth muscle activity, such as that of the colon, and regulate glandular secretion, including digestive juices and hormones. Prostaglandins also control the substances involved in the transmission of nerve impulses, participate in the body's defenses against infection, control fertility, and regulate the rate of metabolism in various tissues. Prostaglandins are major players in causing inflammation and as such, are essential to wellness.

- Vitamin E is a component of many fats and is absolutely necessary to achieve fertility, to avoid cancer, and to maintain a strong immune system. Studies have shown that vitamin E lowers the risk of asthma and allergies, can protect against prostate cancer, and is an essential nutrient in the body's process of calcium absorption.

- CLA, or conjugated linoleic acid, is a fat found in beef and dairy fat. It may be one of our most potent defenses against cancer. In animal studies, as little as one half of one percent CLA in the diet has reduced tumor burden by more than 50 percent. In addition, recent research has shown CLA to decrease abdominal fat, enhance muscle growth, lower insulin resistance, enhance immunity, and reduce food-induced allergic reactions. (For a fuller discussion of the benefits of CLA, read the following section on dairy products.)

- Butyric Acid is a fat found only in dairy products. It is the main food source for the tissues of the colonic mucosa. Butyric fatty acid may be the key ingredient missing in the diet of people who struggle with any form of bowel disturbance from chronic constipation to Irritable Bowel Syndrome

(For a fuller discussion of the benefits of butyric acid, read the following section on dairy products.)

FYI: Butter oil is deep-yellow butter from cows feeding on rapidly growing green grass in the Spring and Fall. Weston Price discovered that butter oil contains vitamins A and D as well as the X Factor.

- Fats affect the nerves. Low-fat diets contribute to depression. The brain is made of fat. There is a high-fat diet used by the medical community to control seizures. This diet consists of 80% fat and is known to work better than drugs.

- Even though this list is long, it is only a small window into the role of healthy fats and oils in the human body. The subject of healthy fat truly deserves an entire book, and more. However, for now I cannot impress upon you enough the importance of fats in the diet. Now, let's take a look at the nutrient-rich traditional fats which have nourished healthy population groups for thousands of years:

  - Butter

  - Beef and lamb tallow

  - Lard

  - Chicken, goose, and duck fat

  - Coconut, palm and sesame oils

  - Cold-pressed olive oil

  - Cold pressed flax oil

  - Marine oils such as cod liver oil

  - Eggs from both birds and reptiles

  - Insects with a fat content as high as 67%

- Am I going to ask you to eat insects? No. But I am going to ask you to go against the voices all around you and eat heaps of fats.

- Even though fats are a nourishing food, there are fats that are damaging to the human body. The following newly used fats (or fats of modern commerce) are not to be used in the diet, as they will cause many health imbalances over time. These imbalances can include but are not limited to cancer, heart dis-

FYI: The Winter 2004 edition of the Weston A. Price magazine called *Wise Traditions* contained an article called "The Quest for Nutrient Dense Food— High Brix Farming and Gardening." Written by WAPF chapter leader Suze Fisher, the article is an interview with Rex Harrill of Keedysville, Maryland. Brix is a measure of nutrient density in plants that is useful for both farmers and consumers. Look for FYI notes in the next several pages about Brix.

ease, immune system dysfunction, sterility, learning disabilities, growth problems and osteoporosis.

- All hydrogenated oils such as margarine

- Soy, corn, and safflower oils

- Cottonseed oil

- Canola oil

- All fats heated to very high temperatures in processing and frying

- Bleached and deodorized oils

These fats are unhealthy for many reasons. One of the main reasons is because they often contain trans-fatty acids. Trans-fat is an unsaturated fat that occurs naturally in low levels in milk and beef. However, 80 percent of the trans-fat Americans consume is from partially hydrogenated vegetable oil found in margarine, packaged baked goods and restaurant fried foods.

- Until around 1990, trans-fat was considered harmless by most. Then studies started to appear that established that trans-fat increases "bad" cholesterol, or LDL, reduces blood vessel function by a third, and lowers "good" blood cholesterol, or HDL. Now that we are certain that trans-fat increases the risk of heart disease, the United States Government has mandated that food manufacturers disclose the amount of trans-fats on food labels by 2006.

- The view that fats, other than vegetable oils, are foods that cause disease has also been shaped by the way in which the animals that our fat sources come from have been raised. The fat from meat from grain-fed animals is high in the omega-6 fatty acid, which is a main culprit in cancer and heart disease. The fat in meat from pastured animals has at least two to four times more omega-3 fatty acids than meat from grain-fed animals and much less omega-6. Omega-3s are formed in the chloroplasts of green leaves and algae, which pasture-fed animals eat. Sixty percent of the fatty acids in grass are omega-3s.

- Products from grass-fed animals offer us more than omega-3 fatty acids. They contain significant amounts of two "good" fats, monounsaturated oils and stearic acid, but no man-made trans-fatty acids. They are also the richest known natural source of CLA and contain extra amounts of vitamin E. The meat from pastured cattle is four times higher in vitamin E than the meat from feedlot cattle and, interestingly, almost twice as high as the meat from feedlot cattle given vitamin E supplements. In humans, vitamin E is linked with a lower risk of heart disease and cancer. This potent antioxidant may also have anti-aging properties. Most Americans are deficient in vitamin E.

- When chickens are housed indoors and deprived of greens, bugs, and worms, both their meat and eggs become artificially low in omega-3 fatty acids. Eggs have provided mankind with high-quality protein and fat-soluble vitamins for thousands of years. Eggs from pastured hens can contain as much as 10 times more omega-3s than eggs from factory hens. Properly produced eggs are rich in just about every nutrient we have yet discovered, especially fat-soluble vitamins A and D. Eggs also provide sulphur-containing proteins, which are necessary for the integrity of cell membranes. Eggs are an excellent source of special long-chain fatty acids called EPA and DHA, which play a vital role in the development of the nervous system in the infant and the maintenance of metal acuity in the adult. With this in mind, it is no wonder that Asians value eggs as a brain food. Egg yolk is the most concentrated source known of choline, a B vitamin found in lecithin that is necessary for keeping the cholesterol moving in the blood stream.

- Our beliefs toward our own body's need for fat in today's world is a prime example of the way in which the market, or capitalism, determines our thinking about what foods we ought to be eating. It is interesting to note that when the dramatic change in fat and oil consumption came to be in the United

FYI: A Brix test requires a hand-held refractometer or Brix meter that contains a prism and an etched scale calibrated in 0-30 or 0-32 degrees Brix. To take a Brix measurement, a consumer or farmer places a few drops of sap (juice) from a plant on the prism. As Rex Harrill (who is interviewed in the *Wise Traditions* article mentioned on the previous page) explains, "Just as a pencil appears bent when placed in a beaker of water, the light passing through the plant juice is bent so that a clear line is shown against the scaled background. The amount of bending is directly related to the richness of the plant juice."

States, the "experts" did not advise us to switch to a low-fat diet like the Japanese, nor to use monounsaturated oils like the Greeks or Italians. Instead, we were advised to replace saturated fat with polyunsaturated oils—primarily corn oil and safflower oil. Cheap corn gave us cheap beef, cheap sugar, and cheap margarine. There have been no people in the history of this planet that have ever eaten large amounts of polyunsaturated oils. However, the experts deemed eating these oils "the right thing to do." Why? The United States had far more corn fields than olive groves, so it seemed reasonable to use the type of oil that we had in abundance

- It is challenging for many to face the fact that we have been lied to for most of our lives. Fats are one of our most important nutrients. Fats are not something to fear but rather to cherish. The lies that fat causes health problems are in place solely to make a profit, and not to intentionally hurt or help people.

Food With High Enzyme Content

Essential Guideline:
Eat foods that are high in enzyme content, including:

- Raw dairy

- Raw meat

- Raw honey

- Tropical fruits such as papaya, pineapple and mango

- Lacto-fermented foods and drinks that are high in bacteria content, such as yogurt, kefir, raw cultured vegetables, and kvass.

Additional Details:

- As we know, as Dr. Price studied the diets of different cultures, he came to appreciate a concept that is very relevant here. He writes in *Nutrition and Physical Degeneration*, "...if the primitive races have been more efficient than modernized groups in the matter of preventing degenerative processes, physical, mental and moral, it is only because they have been more efficient in complying with Nature's Laws." What does this mean, following Nature's Laws? Of course, as we have seen in the previous sections on the importance of high-quality protein and fats, particularly of the animal variety, what Dr. Price thought of as following nature's laws was to give the body what it needed in body-building and body-repairing materials. In other words, following Nature's Laws can mean that we eat only those foods that optimize our bodily functions. By discussing the foods that are high in enzymes and bacteria content, we will learn further what the human body truly needs for optimal health.

- Enzymes are the primary motivators of all natural biochemical processes. Life cannot exist without enzymes because they are essential components of every chemical reaction in the body. In the 1930s, Edward Howell, MD, the food enzyme pioneer, found that there is a difference between enzymes in foods and enzymes that are produced by the body. He was convinced that enzymes in food have a different function in human digestion than that of the body's own digestive enzymes. With this theory, he began isolating and concentrating enzymes from their sources. He found the difference to be that food enzymes begin digesting food in the stomach and will work for at least one hour before the body's digestive system begins to work. In other words, the enzymes in foods assist us to utilize all the nutrients within the foods that we are eating so that none of the food that we eat overworks our bodies. Food is not nourishment to the body if the food is not absorbed by the cells but rather goes along the digestive tract undigested.

> *"When we consume a meal made up entirely of cooked food neither the salivary enzymes nor the upper-stomach enzymes are capable of completing digestion. Foods can then putrefy in the digestive system, and dangerous, health-threatening residues are released into the bloodstream. Under these circumstances, the liver, pancreas, and intestines are constantly overworked. Thus eating most of your food in a cooked state causes undernourished cells, an intestinal tract full of unhealthy bacteria,*

FYI: Low nutrient foods rob the body of nutrients. Rex Harrill also explains this in the *Wise Traditions* article mentioned in the previous pages. He explains, "When our system expends minerals, energy and enzymes to break down food that doesn't even have enough value to replace what is expended, we will lose the battle for life at some point."

Exercise is an
important part of health
maintenance. For many
people, walking is the
perfect exercise. It does
not require athletic ability,
it is very low-risk, and it
puts minimal stress on the
body. Brisk walking:

- Releases endorphins
- Lowers blood pressure
- Burns off calories
- Improves circulation
- Lowers blood sugar in
  diabetics
- Improves memory
- Prevents and reverses
  osteoporosis
- Is inexpensive
- Can be shared with a
  friend
- Produces a sense of
  well-being

a circulation system full of allergens and organs that can not renew themselves.

Total Breast Health
Robin Kenueke

- Raw foods are full of enzymes. A truly healthy diet consists of enzyme-rich foods daily. If a diet doesn't, it isn't a healthy diet. Of course, there are many other guidelines for what constitutes a health-promoting diet, but without ingesting the enzymes from foods, you can not be optimally healthy and live out your longevity potential, and most likely cannot fully recover from an illness. A primary reason for this is that the

---

How Much Fat Should We Eat Per Day?

An excellent guide to how much fat comes from the book, *The Fourfold Path of Healing*, by Thomas Cowan, M. D. expertly incorporated a weighty chapter on nutrition written by Sally Fallon. In this book, Sally Fallon writes a chapter encouraging people to eat as much as 11 tablespoons of saturated, monounsaturated, and polyunsaturated fat each and every day. She writes:

"We are all familiar with the USDA food pyramid, which suggests whole and refined grains as the basis of our diet, with smaller amounts of fruits and vegetables, and very small amounts of animal foods and fats. This is not a concept we endorse-it results in a diet too high in carbohydrates and deficient in saturated fatty acids and the nutrients found exclusively in animals foods. Instead, we propose a different pyramid, one that will provide guidelines for fat consumption. The basis of our pyramid is saturated fats from animal foods and tropical oils. The middle band represents moderate amounts of monounsaturated fatty acids while the peak represents small amounts of polyunsaturated oils."

- The Fourfold Path of Healing,
Thomas Cowan, M.D.

---

body's enzyme potential is depleted when you don't eat raw meats and fats, which in turn drains the body of energy needed to maintain and repair cells, tissues, and organ systems.

- Raw foods were a part of every one of the cultures that Weston A. Price studied. Whether these cultures ate raw food because they understood its importance or because they developed their tastes before they became aware of fire, raw foods were a central food in all traditional fare.

- Many of the raw foods that these earlier cultures ate were from animals—grubs, raw milk, raw organ meats, and the like. Our culture trades the benefits of enzymes for the benefits of profitable foods.

- Many raw foods have a very short shelf-life. Because of this, it has been next to impossible to have a whole array of profitable foods that are provided as raw foods. In addition, raw foods, particularly raw dairy and raw meats, need to be of the highest quality. Meat from animals that are raised for high profit is not meat that can be eaten raw. The chances of meat produced solely for profit and not for health carrying unhealthy bacteria and diseases, such as E coli and Mad Cow Disease, are high. However, raw meat from pastured animals can be eaten raw.

- Because the responsibility of safe food now falls on the consumer and not the supplier, we have all been taught to be afraid of most foods eaten raw. Even the alternative health movement has fallen prey to erroneously negative attitudes toward raw meat created by our food suppliers. Dr. Max Gerson, who established the Gerson Cancer Treatment, had all of his clients eat not only raw vegetable juices but also raw liver. Today, raw liver is no longer a part of the Gerson program due to the powerful fear tactics of the meat industry and the Food and Drug Administration.

- Raw vegetables are less important to our health than raw animal products due to the fact that the proteins and fats in the animal products are our medicinal healing nutrients. These nutrients are always damaged when they are cooked. When

FYI: I use essential oils as implants in colonic therapy, but they also have many other uses. Aromatherapy is a holistic treatment using botanical oils made from plants. Oils can be used to alleviate tension and fatigue, relieve pain, and invigorate the body, or for skin care. When inhaled, essential oils work on the brain and the nervous system through stimulation of the olfactory nerves.

vegetables are cooked, they are more easily digested. It is the heat-sensitive, fat-soluble vitamins, as we saw in the fats and oil section, that are most harmed when one heats or processes the foods from which these health-giving nutrients come in. Furthermore, heat breaks down vitamins and amino acids and produces undesirable cross-linkages in proteins, particularly in meat. Heating meats for more than 3 minutes over 117 degrees Fahrenheit causes proteins to coagulate, denatures the protein molecular structure, leading to deficiency of some essential amino acids and generates numerous carcinogens, including acrolein, nitrosamines, hydrocarbons, and benzopyrene (one of the most potent cancer-causing agents known).

- Heat destroys enzymes. In order to be healthy, you need to ingest lipase, the fat-splitting enzyme, on a daily basis. For those who are struggling with a chronic illness, you cannot be well without therapeutic amounts of lipase; some people may need as much as one pound of raw, pastured butter daily. Lipase allows fat to travel into the places where it promotes health and not illness or obesity. Given that in a real sense, we are entirely cellular membranes, this work of getting fat into the cells where it belongs is incredibly crucial to optimal health. Lipase is responsible for our energy metabolism, the structural integrity of our cells, breaking down lecithin and cholesterol, keeping our bodies free of cancer, and keeping our skin vibrant. Breast milk has a tremendous amount of lipase. For these reasons, raw, pasture-raised butter and high-fat, raw milk are some of our most medicinal foods.

- Fermented foods are an ancient way of preparing and preserving foods that Weston A. Price found practiced in all of the cultures he studied. Microorganisms within fermented foods break down the proteins and the carbohydrates, increasing the digestibility of the food. This increased digestibility assists the body in its cycle of getting required nutrients into the cells.

- Fermented foods are so beneficial to overall health that some of these foods are now considered to be medicines, or "probiotics." The microorganisms in our bodies are largely responsible for our intestinal immune barrier, which keeps harmful materials from entering into our bodies. This barrier is a main component in keeping humans resistant to many diseases, including cancer. Our intestinal microorganisms need to be replenished. This is where fermented foods or foods high in microorganisms come in.

- Within fermented dairy products such as clabbered milk, kefir and yogurt, the lactic acid produced by fermentation of lactose acts as a digestive antiseptic (meaning that it destroys unhealthy bacteria) and a tonic to the nerves of the intestinal tract. This fermentation in raw dairy products also renders calcium, nitrogen, iron, phosphorus, and even fats more available for absorption.

- We no longer have easy access to fermented foods because commercial food-processing techniques have traded many of the benefits of fermented foods for the convenience of mass-produced foods. Traditionally, pickles, olives, sauerkraut, ketchup, and the like were all rich in healthy microorganisms. Today, they are no longer full of these health-giving organisms because fermentation is an inconsistent process, much more of an art than a science, and thus, not profitable. If you leave a jar of fermenting pickles at room temperature on a grocery market shelf, they will continue to ferment and produce CO_2, possibly blowing off the lid or exploding the jar.

- Because of this, most traditionally fermented foods are simply treated with lye to remove the bitterness, and are packed in salt and canned, such as most canned California-style black olives. Olive producers can now hold olives in salt-free brines by using an acidic solution of lactic acid, acetic acid, sodium benzoate and potassium sorbate, a long way off from the old-time natural lactic-acid fermenting method of salt alone.

- All commercial dairy is pasteurized, thereby killing all the healthy bacteria inherent in the milk. In addition, many yogurts are so laden with sugar that the nutritional value has been lost. Unfortunately, such modern techniques as pasteurization effectively kill off all the lactic acid-producing bacteria and short-circuit their important and traditional contribution to intestinal

FYI: The following essential oils are helpful for relieving stress:

Lavender
Rosemary
Geranium
Chamomile
Clary sage
Sandalwood
Juniper berry
Sweet marjoram

and overall health. It is this lactic acid that is so key to the medicinal qualities of fermented dairy products. For many, lactic acid is the only food that resolves chronic constipation, Candida albicans, IBS, Crohn's disease, chronic mood imbalances, and so on.

- You can still find some healthy traditional varieties of fermented foods. The stronger-flavored, traditional Greek olives you are most likely to find on olive bars are not lye-treated and are still alive with active cultures. So are "overnights," the locally crocked fresh pickling cucumbers made in local delis every few days. Olives, sauerkraut, pickles, yogurt, clabbered milk and kefir are all easily made at home. In order to learn how to make these medicinal foods, see our recipe section at the end of this book, and do read through Sally Fallon's book, *Nourishing Traditions* for her numerous recipes for fermented foods.

- I recommend starting out with one tablespoon of any fermented product and building from there. It is important to start slowly with fermented food products because of their influences on the levels of healthy to unhealthy bacteria in the intestinal ecosystem.

Soups Prepared With Bone Broths

Essential Guideline:
Eat soup that has been prepared using soup bones.
Each and every one of the cultures that Dr. Price studied used bones to make soup broth.

Additional Details:

- Most of us know the healing value of a good soup. The only problem, as with almost all foods, is that the nourishing side of soup has been traded in for convenience so that there is almost no soup on the grocery store shelf that is optimally healthy.

- Using bones to make soup makes calcium more available to the body and easier to assimilate. In addition, these soups are rich in sodium, chloride, magnesium, phosphorus, potassium, and sulphur in a ready-to-use ionized form as a true electrolyte solution.

- Using bones to make soup makes certain proteins like proline and glycine more digestible. These amino acids work together to build and to maintain strong bones and cartilage. In addition, these amino acids give nourishment to the skin, the digestive tract, the immune system, the heart, and the muscles. Using bones to make soups provides us with gelatin. Most of us know about Jell-O. This food is a classic example of what has happened to most of our traditionally nourishing foods. Gelatin has become Jell-O, a "tasty," sugar- and MSG-laden food, instead of a food that is nutrient-dense. Gelatin-rich broths help to detoxify the liver, and they aid in digestion by making the foods within the soup more easily digested. I recommend that you eat soup made with bones one time per day while you are working through Ten Days to Optimal Health.

<aside>
FYI: High sugar intake in the diet not only contributes to hyperglycemia (high blood sugar), but it is also linked to heart disease, diabetes, and free radical stress from the oxidation of glucose. Glucose oxidizes much faster than fat.
</aside>

Raw Dairy

Essential Guideline:
Eat raw dairy products.

Additional Details:

- Since the beginnings of our current system of modern medicine, we have been encouraged to use food as medicine. Hippocrates, the most famous of all physicians, contended that nature has an innate power to heal, and the quotation, "Let your food be your medicine, and your medicine be your food" is attributed to him. He recommended milk and its products as wonderful foods.

- D2, which is the vitamin D that commercial dairy products are fortified with, is not the vitamin D that naturally occurs in milk, but rather one of many D components that our bodies need. If you look at the labels of most packaged foods, you will find that the foods are fortified. These vitamins and minerals are not the nutrients that your body needs to be optimally healthy.

- Traditionally, all cultures ate freely of organ meat, fish, shellfish, birds, reptiles, insects, dairy foods and/or red meat. As a result of this diet, our ancestors had four times the calcium and other minerals and ten times the fat-soluble vitamins A and D as we do today. In addition, our ancestors consumed large quantities of Activator X and the Wulzen factor. What are

---

The Intestinal Ecosystem: The Missing Link

Declining levels of healthy bacteria in most people's intestinal tracts, due to not only a lack of fermented foods in the diet, but also to an overuse of antibiotics, a lack of locally grown, organic food in the diet, and an excessive consumption of carbohydrates, all encourages an overgrowth of toxin-producing organisms such as Candida albicans and Clostridium species. These naturally occurring organisms then overpopulate the intestinal tract and cause a wide array of confusing health problems. When these naturally occurring organisms are overgrown in our bodies, they become opportunistic parasites. Most of us are overrun with these parasites. Because of this, our bodies are vulnerable to many health problems. Some of these problems are:

a) A microbial overgrowth can cause structural damage to the intestinal mucosa, thereby diminishing its ability to eliminate waste and maintain a blood barrier for microbial and dietary waste. This condition is called "leaky gut," and leads to many autoimmune diseases and food allergies.

b) The waste products of many of these organisms are toxic. These toxic wastes place an increased load on the body.

Many people then become allergic to their own inner environment, which turns into chronic illness, chemical sensitivities, fibromyalgia, irritable bowel, and so on. Crohn's disease, which afflicts more than 500,000 people in the United States, is a classic example of a person's immune system trying to deal with an overload of microbes. Because our microbes are very much a "part" of our tissues, the immune system is forced to attack the body's own tissues in an attempt to remove the excess microbes and their toxins.

c) The enzymes from some of these bacteria convert normal stool, derived from food and bile, into chemicals that can cause cancer. Given that microbial overgrowth tends to be pervasive in modern living, it is no wonder that colon cancer is the number-two occurring cancer in this country.

d) Chronic fatigue, mood disorders, skin problems, obesity, diabetes, and GERD, all have as one of their causes a microbial overgrowth.

e) Constipation is largely caused by an overgrowth of unhealthy microbes. Stool is largely the byproduct of the life cycle of healthy bacteria. When a colon is overgrown with unhealthy microbes, it is almost impossible for the body to produce a healthy, daily bowel movement.

FYI: Cell membranes in our bodies have a need for both omega 6 and omega 3. The ideal ratio is five omega 6 to one omega 3. Unfortunately, the typical American diet has 15 to 20 omega 6 to one omega 3. Fish-based omega 3 fatty acid in the form of cod liver oil is a helpful source of this necessary nutrient.

these? Without these nutrients, your body cannot—absolutely cannot—fully use any of the other excellent nutrients from the foods that you are eating.

• Raw dairy foods from grass-fed cows may be our healthiest source of nourishment at this point in history. Most of us are not going to eat organ meats or insects. Most of our fish is contaminated with mercury and other toxins. Raw, grassfed, dairy is high in enzymes, vitamin A, vitamin D, and Activator X, along with many other nutrients. Even if you have an excellent diet, if you don't have these nutrients in high enough quantity, you will not absorb your fats, your minerals, or your water-soluble vitamins.

- True vitamin A, or retinol, is found only in animal products like free-range eggs, cod liver oil, liver and other organ meats, insects, fish, shellfish, and butterfat from cows eating green grass. Your most easily absorbed source of vitamin A is butterfat from raw butter and raw cream. Vitamin A from animal sources is not the same as its precursors, namely the carotenes found in plant foods. The conversion of carotenes in the human body is often compromised, and even under optimal conditions is not efficient enough to supply the amount of true vitamin A that Price found in the diets of healthy isolated populations.

- One particular important nutritional constituent of dairy foods that is central to the work of cleansing, and especially rebuilding of the intestinal tract, is a fatty acid called *butyrate*. Butyrate is the preferred fuel for the cells in the large-intestine mucosa, and is a modulator of immune response and inflammation in the colon. The only source of butyrate in our diet is from cow's milk. There are a number of scientific studies suggesting that butyrate is useful in reducing symptoms and restoring colon health in ulcerative colitis. Many doctors claim that their clients are helped with butyrate enemas. Butyrate levels are commonly measured in comprehensive stool analyses, and they act as a marker for levels of beneficial bacteria.

- Butyrate, found in cow's milk, has been shown to significantly inhibit the growth of cancerous colon cells. Scientists have long linked butyrate levels in the colon to overall reductions in the incidence of colon cancer. It is thought that butyrate affects a chemical that slows the growth of cancer cells. Butyric acid can also modify colonic cells, and in the case of cancerous colonic cells overcomes their resistance to normal programmed death. Thus, the activities of butyrate may contribute substantially to a decreased incidence of bowel cancer.

- CLA, or conjugated linoleic acid, is a type of fat that may prove to be one of our most potent cancer fighters. In laboratory animals, a very small percentage of CLA—a mere 0.1 percent of total calories—greatly reduced tumor growth. In a Finnish study, women who had the highest levels of CLA in their diet had a 60 percent lower risk of breast cancer than those with the lowest levels.

- Milk from a pastured cow can have five times as much CLA as a grain-fed animal. Switching from grain-fed to grass-fed dairy products places women in this lowest risk category.

- Pasture-grazed cows have 500% more CLA in their milk than those fed silage.

> "The discovery of CLA in the fat of grass-fed ani-
> mals—in butterfat, tallow, and suet—and the emerg-
> ing revelations as to its benefits, has posed an embar-
> rassing dilemma for apologists of the factory farming
> system. Scientists are looking for feed supplements
> that induce confinement cows to produce CLA and for
> ways to produce CLA in the laboratory so it can be
> sold in supplement form. The solution, of course, is to
> phase out confinement feeding and put cows back on
> green pasture where they belong."
>
> - Jo Robinson
> Pasture Perfect

FYI: Farm-raised fish may have less mercury than fish exposed to our water supplies, but they are fed corn and other foods that lack Omega 3 fatty acid. The tanks that are used to grow fish also contain toxic levels of PCBs.

- The benefits of a diet high in calcium cannot be understated. We can see through the work of Weston Price and through many archeological studies that historically, people have eaten calcium rich diets. This history of a calcium-rich diet is still within our genes. We need lots of calcium in our day-to-day diet. Not only is calcium vital for strong bones and teeth, but it's also needed for the heart, the nervous system and for muscle growth and contraction.

- Even with all the media attention on our need for calcium, especially women's need for calcium, we still struggle with high levels of diseases that are caused in part by a lack of sufficient calcium in the diet.

- Both cancer and osteoporosis are diseases reflective of a calcium deficiency. Why is this? Again, it has to do with the quality of the calcium available to most of us. Calcium carbonate, the most common form of calcium in supplements, is chalk. This is not what our bodies are looking for. Calcium in meats, vegetables, and grains are difficult to absorb. Both iron and zinc can inhibit calcium absorption, as can excess phosphorus and magnesium. Phytic acid in the bran of grains that have not been soaked, fermented, sprouted, or naturally leavened will bind with calcium in the intestinal tract, making calcium less absorbable.

- Sufficient vitamin D, which is lacking in commercial dairy products is needed for calcium absorption. Sugar consumption and stress both pull calcium from the bones.

- The best sources of usable calcium are dairy products and bone broth. In cultures where dairy products are not used, bone broth is essential.

- Lactose, or milk sugar, is the most important carbohydrate for the colon flora. Just as yogurt or kefir-making bacteria thrive off the lactose in milk, so do our own internal bacteria thrive with lactose. If you really want to keep your intestine full of healthy bacteria, drink at least one cup daily of raw milk from pasture-raised cows or goats.

- You cannot be healthy without an adequate dietary intake of lipase. Raw milk products are a tasty and easy way to ingest large quantities of lipase.

- Of course, it is crucial that the farmer assures the healthfulness of the cow's milk by assuring the health of the cow. Historically, this has not been done, which is why raw milk has gotten such a bad name. Raw milk is a safe food. It has been commercially available in California for decades, with not a single adverse affect.

- Raw milk is inherently safe. Microbiologist Lee Dexter says that raw milk not only is safe, but may be healthier than pasteurized milk. The former USDA employee sells raw goat's milk in Texas, where it is legal. Lee Dexter has reviewed numerous cases worldwide and has written a lengthy report on raw milk. She said most comments made by epidemiologists and public health officials on the dangers of raw milk are opinions and "are not based on scientific fact." She said statistics from the Centers for Disease Control and Prevention clearly show that "people drinking pasteurized milk are four times more likely to contract a food-borne illness" than those who drink raw milk. Dexter said "challenge tests," in which raw milk was inoculated with pathogens and examined later, showed that the pathogens were destroyed. "Raw milk contains its own immune system," she said.

FYI: Although foods such as yogurt, sauerkraut, and kefir are available in developed countries, they are pasteurized, processed, and modified so that they no longer provide the same health benefits.

My Personal Experience With Raw Dairy Products

My passion and my clinical understanding of raw dairy bring to my mind a personal story. Remember that I had been very sick for years, even when I was eating "perfectly," healing emotionally, and living the most healthful lifestyle I could come up with—asleep by ten, playing the piano, colon cleansing, sleeping in air conditioning to minimize my mold exposure, and so on. I never "cheated." I hated being sick. When I was symptomatic, I always thought that I was going to die. I do not want to die young. Forty is young. Fifty is young. Sixty is young. I am fully determined to live beyond 100.

When my primary health-care practitioner suddenly died of cancer, I was lost. One month before, I had sat with her in her office. She "seemed" in good health. As she always did, she took a look at my urine and saliva pH, asked me what I was eating, and, accordingly, adjusted my supplements and diet. Even though I followed her direction diligently for 3 years, I was still symptomatic every day. But I was neither bedridden nor bleeding from my colon. When she died, I cried my eyes out for three days. Once I had overcome some of the pain of her death, I was able to start thinking about what to do next.

FYI: In the early to mid-20th century, German researchers documented kombucha as an intestinal regulator that benefits digestive disturbances, constipation, hemorrhoids, kidney stones, gall bladder problems, diabetes, cholesterol, high blood pressure, angina, gout, eczema, arthritis, rheumatism, atherosclerosis, irritability, anxiety, headaches, dizziness and fatigue.

Fortunately, I had a friend who had helped me to find healers to work with over the years, so I thought to consult her about what I might do. We decided that Dr. Mercola, who practices close to Madison, WI, USA, was the healer to seek help from. My friend went to see him. When she returned, she said he was excellent, but instead of going to see him, I could learn Metabolic Typing. I have, and it has been my great fortune to study with Dodie Anderson of the Metabolic Typing Education Center.

From day one, Dodie encouraged me to use raw dairy, especially butter, as therapeutic foods. I was resistant, to say the least. All my training told me to avoid all dairy products.

WARNING: Some People May Be Sensitive to Raw Dairy

Some people may be sensitive to raw daiy due to a compromised immune system. Modern man is affected by conditions duch as candida albicans that is caused by medical treatment and indiscrimiate use of antibiotics in agriculture. Whether or not we have taken antibiotics for colds or a skin condition, most of us have eaten meat, poultry and eggs that contain residues of antibiotics from unhealthy agricultural practices. The indigenous populations that Weston A. Price studied were untouched by these practices and had healthy immune systems.

No group is more dedicated to raw dairy than the growing numbers who follow Weston A. Price. However, even among this dedicated group, there are people who cannot eat raw dairy, fermented foods and bone broths due to food sensitivities. Many of these people have been able to slowly add the Weston A. Price foods to their diet and have found that their body adapts over time. To read posts from WAPF chapter leaders on this subject, visit www.onibasu.com. Onibasu is a public search engine that contains an index of the WAPF chapter leaders e-group.

FYI: Sally Fallon's article called "Kvass and Kombucha, Gifts from Russia" may be found at: www.westonprice.org/foodfeatures/kvass.htm

CHAPTER FIVE

What Foods To Avoid and Why

"In our country, however, we see malnutrition as over consumptive and under nutrition, which means that we eat too much of too little."

- Jeffrey Bland Ph.D.
Introductory Nutrition

When you're learning what foods to avoid to stay healthy, think of these fundamental principles:

1. **All grains, nuts, and seeds have enzyme inhibitors and phytic acid that are present in the outer skin or milled product.** This means that all commercial bread, crackers, muffins, pasta, and other products made from these foods put a strain on your digestion. This is also the case with soybean that is a legume. Soy is a heavily promoted food in the United States. Sally Fallon explains that while she was researching phytic acid for her book *Nourishing Traditions*, she kept reading about the high levels of phytic acid in soy. She found:

   • Reports written by the soy industry in the 1970s on how they were trying to get phytic acid and also enzyme inhibitors out of the soy by processing, and how difficult this was to do.

   • The Rackis studies showing the damage to the pancreas of rats consuming processed soy protein in industry-sponsored studies.

   • A quote on how they were going to market soy as a health product to the upscale market, in order to then have it accepted by the general public.

FYI: According to the July 26, 2000 issue of *Journal of the American Medical Association*, doctors are the third leading cause of deaths in the United States.

2. **Starchy vegetables may adversely effect your blood sugar levels.** Indirectly, foods that effect your blood sugar levels can also cause high blood pressure and free-radical stress.

3. **All processed food contains synthetic chemicals that act as preservatives.** Food manufacturers and food retailers are concerned about shelf life. This same principle applied to pasteurized dairy that is heated to high temperatures to kill pathogenic bacteria. Raw dairy is a superior food, but only if you can obtain if from a farmer who has healthy animals. Most dairies—including those that sell pasteurized, organic milk—often have filthy cesspools with cows standing in manure several feet deep. The factory dairy cow is also fed a mash full of antibiotics and hormones such as rBGH, waste products, and even meat from infected animals, even though the cow is an herbivore (vegetarian).

Summary Guide to the "Foods To Avoid" List

Make a copy of the following summary guide of foods to avoid and put it on your refrigerator. Your work with the "to avoid" list will be just as important as the new foods you are adding.

1. Grains
   _____

   Avoid wheat, oats, rye, rice, barley, and all other grains. To do this, you will need to stay away from bread, cookies, muffins, bagels, pasta, tabouli, couscous, and all other grain products.

2. Starchy vegetables
   _____

   Starchy vegetables, including potatoes, squash, corn and popcorn. Vegetables in this category that can be used sparingly include carrots, beets, parsnips, and turnips, as these are good as garnishes and for flavor.

3. Pasteurized dairy
   _____

   Products in this category include yogurt, cream, butter, cheese, cottage cheese, and ice cream.

4. Sweeteners

   Sweeteners to avoid include sugar, honey, maple syrup, brown-rice sweetener, chocolate, corn syrup, and fructose. Read labels, as these are frequently added to packaged goods.

5. Beans or legumes including all soy products.

   For in-depth details about soy, visit www.westonaprice.org

6. Alcohol, coffee, and soda.

   It is best to avoid these beverages during your nutrition program.

7. Processed foods, preservatives, artificial ingredients, or additives.

   One of the most important ingredients to avoid in this category is MSG. Celtic sea salt is a healthy ingredient and may be consumed liberally.

8. Processed, smoked, or commercially produced meats.

   This category includes farm-raised fish.

Grains

Essential Guideline:
Avoid wheat, oats, rye, rice, barley, and all other grains.

Additional Details:

- Grains are central to many health problems. The neat thing about the OHC Plan is that it is a simple test to find out how you feel when you eat or don't eat different foods and let your body tell you what works best. Many people find that grains cause health problems. That is no surprise since we were not genetically designed to subsist on daily grains. What follows is a small list of what can happen, over time, due to eating grains:

   1) The high phytate content of whole grains tends to interfere with mineral metabolism. An inadequate supply of minerals in the body causes many problems.

FYI: According to Dr. Barbara Starfield of the Johns Hopkins School of Hygiene and Public Health, who wrote an article about the U.S. health care system for the July 26, 2000 issue of the *Journal of the American Medical Association*, the number of deaths per year from iatrogenic causes (induced in a patient by physician activity, manner or therapy) is 250,000.

2) There are substances in grains that have the potential to interact with the gastrointestinal tract and the immune system that can cause what is known as leaky gut, a condition in which the intestinal wall becomes permeable. A permeable gut lets toxins, food particles, and yeast organisms into the peripheral circulation, where they wreak havoc.

3) Grains are high in carbohydrates, which can cause your pancreas to overwork. The pancreas is a large gland located underneath the stomach. In addition to its all-important job of producing insulin to control your blood sugar levels, the pancreas produces a bicarbonate solution with an alkalinity of about 8. This solution plays an important role in neutralizing the chyme acid delivered from the stomach. When reaching for optimal health, it is essential to keep this area of the small intestines slightly alkaline. When the pancreas is overworked, it cannot do its job of producing enough bicarbonate, and this can result in emotional imbalance, elevated cholesterol, weight gain, and disturbed sleep. (For these same reasons, you will be limiting your consumption of starchy vegetables and beans during this plan.)

4) Grains tend to cause unhealthy organisms in your digestive tract, such as yeast, to overgrow. Having an overgrowth state of unhealthy organisms in the digestive tract can lead to very serious complications with a wide variety of symptoms including: gas, bloating, cramping, pain, indigestion, nausea, diarrhea, and constipation. In addition to these digestive difficulties, an overgrowth state often causes bodily problems not typically associated with the colon, such as heart irregularities, numbness, tingling, joint and muscle pain, fatigue, sinus and respiratory problems, chemical sensitivities, hormonal imbalances, headaches, and even vision problems.

• Once you have succeeded in following this 35-day health plan, you may want to add grains back to your diet. However, some people may find that their bodies don't tolerate grains well after not eating them for 35 days. If after eating grains, you find yourself gassy, bloated, and with headaches or any other previous symptom, I would suspect grains. Take them out of your diet for at least three days, and, if you wish, try again. Try them slowly. For instance, you may have one grain serving two days after your fast.

- If after working through this program you decide to include grains in your diet, I highly recommend that you follow the ways of the traditional cultures and soak or ferment your grains. Each culture that Dr. Price studied always soaked or fermented their grains. All grains contain phytic acid.

"Untreated phytic acid can combine with calcium, magnesium, copper, iron, and especially zinc in the intestinal tract and block their absorption. This is why a diet high in unfermented whole grains may lead to serious mineral deficiencies and bone loss. The modern misguided practice of consuming large amounts of unprocessed bran often improves colon transit time at first but may lead to Irritable Bowel Syndrome and, in the long term, many other adverse effects. Soaking allows enzymes, lactobacilli and other helpful organisms to break down and neutralize phytic acid."

- Nourishing Traditions
Sally Fallon

FYI: Lactoperoxidase, a naturally existing enzyme in raw milk, reacts with thiocyanate, which is also naturally found in milk, in the presence of hydrogen peroxide. The resulting compound has a bactericidal effect on bacteria such as Escherichia coli.

Starchy Vegetables

Essential Guideline:
Avoid starchy vegetables, including potatoes, squash, corn, and popcorn.

Additional Details:
- The Glycemic Index (GI) was first developed by Canadian Professor of Nutrition David Jenkins in 1981. It's a tool that is designed to help diabetics control blood sugar It's also helpful for hypoglycemics who need to control their reaction to carbohydrates. Jenkins and his fellow researchers studied how quickly various foods affect blood sugar, and they assigned

The time required
to brew kombucha will
vary depending on the
temperature. Your brewing
will speed up in the sum-
mer and slow down in the
winter.

a numerical value to foods. The value indicates how rapidly
50 grams of a food will raise blood sugar compared to a food
that is known to be rapidly digested (glucose). The researchers
classified foods as follows:

1. High Glycemic Foods
   High glycemic foods (80 and higher) digest rapidly and
   cause a fast release of glucose into the blood stream.

2. Low Glycemic Foods
   Low glycemic foods (40 and lower) digest slowly and
   release glucose into the blood gradually.

Although most of the GI contains values for foods that are not
included in the Weston A. Price diet, the list of vegetables is a
helpful guide for understanding which foods are starchy.

Vegetables Beets	64
Carrots (raw)	31
Carrots (cooked)	36
Corn, sweet	55
Potato (baked)	98
Potato (red skin, boiled)	70
Potato, yams	71
Parsnips	131
Pumpkin	107

Pasteurized Dairy

Essential Guideline:
Avoid pasteurized yogurt, cream, butter, cheese, cottage cheese,
and ice cream.

Additional Details:

- Very few of us can truly digest today's commercial dairy products. The reason for confining our cows in feedlots and feeding
  them grain rather than grass is that they produce more milk—
  especially when injected with biweekly hormones.

- Today's grain-fed cows produce three times as much milk as
  the old family cow of days gone by. The protein in pasteurized

cow's milk is the leading cause of food allergies in both adults and children. The fat in pasteurized and homogenized milk has been altered and no longer comes with the lipase enzyme that is needed by the body to digest the milk fat.

- There is also evidence that pasteurized dairy consumption causes immune-system reactions that trigger arthritis, atherosclerosis, and type I diabetes. Also, numerous studies have linked pasteurized dairy intake to an increased risk of cancer, especially breast cancer. Ask around. You'll be surprised to find how many people have already figured out that giving up pasteurized dairy has decreased the number of colds they get, the sinus problems they have, the number of ear infections their children get, and the amount of bloating they experience.

- Although pasteurized dairy is not a part of this program, raw milk from cows that eat green nutrient-dense grass and has its enzymes intact is an excellent source of nutrients.

FYI: Lipitor, a statin drug that doctors prescribe to lower cholesterol, has serious side effects that include depression, infertility, back pain, muscle weakness, and neuropathy.

Sweeteners

Essential Guideline:
Sweeteners to avoid include sugar, honey, maple syrup, brown rice sweetener, chocolate, corn syrup, and fructose.

Additional Details:

- According to the *Journal of Natural Medicine* (Volume 1, Number 9, page five), 1 teaspoon of refined sugar paralyzes 50 percent of your white blood cells for five hours. And that's if you've had no more than a teaspoon of sugar. Sugar reduces the ability of white blood cells to destroy foreign particles and microorganisms, and this negative effect starts within less than 30 minutes. It lasts for over five hours, and typically your white blood cells show a 50 percent reduction in their ability to destroy and engulf foreign particles. During this time of healing, you especially need those valuable white blood cells to help you cleanse, heal, and strengthen your body. Also, when blood sugar levels rise too rapidly, a message is sent to the intestinal tract to slow down because glucose is absorbed mostly in the first part of the small intestines. When you eat sugar week in and week out, it causes the digestive tract to stop moving.

- Sugar causes the body to become overly acidic. The body cannot function soundly in this pH range. The small intestines and the stomach cannot protect themselves well against the hazards of acid. The small intestines were designed to function in a slightly alkaline environment because the intestinal and pancreatic enzymes work best in a neutral or slightly alkaline environment. In order to regain a healthy balance, our body will use up important alkaline minerals such as calcium, magnesium, and potassium. A common sign of excess acidity due to the consumption of sugar is heartburn. Over time, all bodily systems become worn out.

- If after this program you decide to eat sugar, it will be useful to your body if you know a few facts. Whenever you are eating a food with sugar, you must create a balance to the sugar with large amounts of minerals. Foods made by nature, like an apple or a banana or maple syrup or raw honey, contain minerals along with the sugars. This gives the body its needed tools to effectively metabolize the sugar. A candy bar hasn't the nutrients to assist the body in handling the toxicity of sugar. You must also have an abundance of micro flora living in your digestive tract to both retain minerals in the intestines and to "eat up" those sugars while they are being processed before entering into your blood and your cells. The micro flora are there to process the sugars and still maintain a body in balance.

- During a cleanse, sweets such as honey, brown-rice syrup, molasses, and maple syrup can dramatically upset your blood sugar as well as the ratio of healthy to unhealthy microorganisms in your digestive tract. Your body needs to use its energy to clean house and heal and it will appreciate the break from the exhausting work of metabolizing sweets.

- For the sweet flavor in your diet, which I believe can be crucial to a successful plan, try Stevia or vegetable glycerin instead of granular sugars. Stevia is an herb from South America. It is not toxic like sugar and it works well in tea and in many dessert recipes. Because it does have a bit of an aftertaste, similar to that of artificial sweeteners, it might take some getting used to. The key is to start with a very, very small amount and, if needed, to increase the amount gradually, as Stevia is 200-300 times sweeter than sugar.

- Vegetable glycerin is derived from coconut and is another easy substitute for sugar. It is a clear liquid and works like honey. Glycerin has 80 calories per tablespoon.

- Raw honey can also be an excellent food for many people. However, raw honey is high in carbohydrates and can easily imbalance your blood sugar levels. Until you know your sensitivities to sugars, by following Ten Days to Optimal Health, I do not recommend that you use raw honey. Once you have a greater understanding of your strengths and weaknesses, raw honey may be a nutritious food for you.

Beans or Legumes

Essential Guideline:
Avoid beans and legumes, including all soy products.

Additional Details:

- Soy is a food of modern commerce. It tends to be highly processed and contains lots of phytoestrogens that have negative hormonal effects. People with thyroid problems need to avoid soy altogether. Soy may be a healthy small part of your diet, but not a staple.

- Soy in Asia is normally a fermented food, being processed to remove toxins. And it is usually eaten with meat. In Japan, soy is eaten with fish, and in China, soy is eaten with pork as 1-2% of total calories of the diet. Soy, in very small quantities, may be an excellent food for many.

- During this plan, I recommend that you avoid soy altogether. This will give your body a chance to clear out any soy sensitivity. After this plan, you may or may not want to add soy back into your diet as a fermented food in small amounts.

FYI: Of all foods, milk has the lowest incidence of reported food-born illnesses (.02%).

On a case-by-case basis, persons consuming milk from any source (raw or pasteurized) are:

- 30 times more likely to become ill from fruits and vegetables
- 13 times more likely to become ill from beef
- 11 times more likely to become ill from chicken
- 10 times more likely to become ill from potato salad
- 2.7 times more likely to become ill from non-dairy beverages

  - *Raw Milk and Raw Milk Products* by Lee Dexter, White Egret Farms
  - Sally Fallon, Weston A. Price Foundation

FYI: Your bottled kombucha may form a gelatinous mass. Strain this before drinking.

Alcohol, Coffee and Soda

Essential Guideline:
It is best to avoid these beverages during your nutrition plan.

Additional Details:

- Alcohol contains elements of fermentation that can be dangerously stressful and damaging to the liver, which is our major filter of toxins as well as the major organ of digestion. Alcohol also damages glandular/immune organs, connective tissue, and the nervous system. For those of you who find it hard to give up alcohol, twelve step programs such as Alcoholics Anonymous are welcoming and have healing tools that do work. Your life will be greatly enriched by doing the emotional and spiritual work of the steps. I am a recovering alcoholic, and I am sure that I would be dead today if I hadn't made the decision to give up alcohol and tackle my healing.

- Coffee can be very hard on your body. It makes the body overly acidic, it kills the healthy microbes in your gut, and it tends to throw your blood sugar off balance. Coffee addiction is a sign that your adrenal glands are already exhausted, and coffee drains those glands even more. All of these imbalances make it hard for the body to truly rest, and they make it hard for the individual to know what their limits are. For these reasons, I strongly recommend no coffee or a coffee substitute during the course of the plan.

- Many people find that coffee is almost impossible to give up because it is one of their most important and essential daily rituals. I honor that people need rituals that allow them to feel that life is good, the fact that they can handle the chores of day-to-day life. Unfortunately, for many this contentment comes with their daily cup of coffee. If this is the case with you, you will want to find a coffee substitute like green or herbal tea. With teas, you can really experiment. One of my favorite tea mixtures is raspberry leaf and peppermint. Go out and get yourself a lot of different teas and have fun.

- For some, I permit coffee in the plan during the first ten days, which makes it possible for people to start the process of cleansing and fully nourishing their cells while still having something of a treat. I had tried to give up coffee many times. I knew that drinking coffee made me sick. But each time I tried to give it up, I would get an overwhelming feeling that I had given up all that I loved. I would cry hard, but after a few days I just couldn't stand the loneliness anymore. This went on for a few years. Finally, after doing the emotional work, I figured out that I had started drinking caffeinated beverages just about the time that my 13 year-old brother had been violently killed by a car while riding his bike. By giving up coffee, I was pulling up the painful emotions attached to the loss of my brother that I hadn't yet cleared out. Through this process of giving up the coffee and grieving the loss of the coffee, I have been able to more fully heal from the death of my brother. Now I am coffee free, more connected to the people in my life who are still alive and incredibly pleased about it. Do use these places where you are emotionally attached to foods and drinks to heal from the hurts of your life. You will be amazed at how much of yourself you recover from the past.

- If needed, tackle this no-coffee recommendation in the second or third ten-day cycle. And as you go, do take my recommendations and set up some time for yourself to have a full-out tantrum about how much you want coffee. Making adaptations to a healthy lifestyle, which will work for you in reaching your goals over the long haul, is always a smart idea.

- Besides the sugar or the NutraSweet in soda, studies demonstrate that phosphorus, a frequent ingredient of soda, can deplete bones of calcium. Phosphorus, which occurs naturally in some foods and is used as an additive in many others, appears to weaken bones by promoting the loss of calcium throughout the entire body. With less calcium available, the bones suffer by becoming more porous and prone to fractures, and osteoporosis.

FYI: Dutch researchers found much lower rates of Salmonella infections in dairy herds and cows with access to pasture.

- *Raw Milk and Raw Milk Products* by Lee Dexter, White Egret Farms
- Sally Fallon, Weston A. Price Foundation

Processed Food, Preservatives, and Artificial Ingredients or Additives

Essential Guideline:
One of the most important ingredients to avoid in this category is MSG. Celtic sea salt is a healthy ingredient and may be consumed liberally.

Additional Details:

• Each year the FDA approves more and more chemicals for use in foods. These chemicals increase shelf life, kill bacteria, improve taste, replace fats, replace carbohydrates, and replace protein. This is insane. Many of us now eat chemicals for our nourishment instead of vital macronutrients. To our food suppliers, profit is the key factor in food production. Unfortunately, for the consumer of these fancy foods, food additives are often neurotoxic and/ or carcinogenic. Thousands of the processed foods on the market are loaded with synthetic chemicals, which inside your body overload your organs of elimination. These chemicals are then stored in your cells, where they cause damage. Where the chemicals are stored is different in every individual. This is why one person might end up with cancer and another with irritable bowel.

• One particularly harsh and ubiquitous chemical is MSG, or monosodium glutamate. It is used in very large amounts in processed food due to the fact that it adds flavor and is addictive. Do not eat it. For one thing, it will increase your chances of obesity. In addition, scientific studies have shown it to permanently shift neural mechanisms in your brain that will alter your mood. Unfortunately, the foods that contain it are not usually labeled as having MSG. Restaurants often use it in their dishes. Always ask the wait staff and cook when you go out to eat, and request that they don't add MSG to your dish, or for that matter, to anyone's dish.

• Table salt is hard on your body because it is highly refined by drying it at over 1,200 degrees Fahrenheit. This amount of heat changes the chemical structure of the salt. Also, conventional processing adds harmful additives and chemicals, such as lead,

Fragrances, Volatile Chemicals and Cigarettes
Chemicals in the environment are poisonous to our bodies as much as the chemicals in food.

1. Fragrances and volatile chemicals
Perfumes, including scented soaps for your body and hands, colognes, underarm deodorants, aftershaves, shampoos, hair conditioners, and almost all house cleaning products, laundry detergents, and dryer sheets contain fragrances that are volatile chemicals that poison your liver, lungs, kidneys, bladder, adrenals, and nervous system. They invade the body and those around you by the chemicals' direct access to the bloodstream through the mucous membranes of the respiratory passages. This toxic cycle forces your detoxification system to work overtime.

2. Cigarettes
The smoke from a cigarette exposes your body to over 600 dangerous chemicals, including heavy metals such as cadmium, formaldehyde, phenol, acetaldehyde, and arsenic. Smoking while on this program is obviously counterproductive to the work that you are trying to accomplish. The great news is that within two weeks most of the nicotine will be gone from your body. Yes, it only takes two weeks for the majority of nicotine to leave your body. By the end of this program, you can easily be a nonsmoker. And this program is set up to make it much easier to quit smoking. Bile, from the gallbladder, is your main tool for carrying the nicotine and other toxins out of your body in these two weeks. Colon cleansing, and particularly coffee enemas, increase the flow of bile out of your body. Thus, if you are quitting smoking, take coffee enemas, after your cleansing enemas, one to seven times per week. Once the nicotine is out of the body, all physical withdrawal will cease.

During the initial two weeks and after, it is important to realize that stress has a physiological effect on the body,

FYI: Consumers are avoiding commercial milk not only because it is pasteurized, but also because it comes mostly from cows kept in confinement, a situation that encourages poor health and disease (confinement cows live an average of 42 months versus 12-15 years for a cow on pasture).

- *Raw Milk and Raw Milk Products* by Lee Dexter, White Egret Farms
- Sally Fallon, Weston A. Price Foundation

FYI: Use a plastic straw to test your kombucha (push the straw down into the brew and hold your thumb over one end of the straw to draw out some liquid).

which increases the desire for cigarettes. Stress makes the urine acidic. Whenever the urine becomes acidic, the body excretes more nicotine. Thus, when a smoker encounters a stressful situation, he excretes more nicotine and goes into withdrawal.

Most smokers feel that when they are nervous or upset, cigarettes help calm them down. The calming effect from cigarettes is not relief from the emotional strain of a situation, but actually the effect of replenishing the nicotine supply and ending the withdrawal. During stressful times, take more coffee enemas. During stressful times, find a friend who can listen to you rant and rave about the stressful situation. During stressful times, play a musical instrument. During stressful times, take a long walk in a favorite spot and cry. And do try to diminish the amount of stress that you are under when you take on quitting smoking. And it is fine to take on quitting smoking a week or two into the program. Always remember that your goal is to be successful. With small and steadfast steps, you will be successful!

aluminum, and mercury. This processing of the salt strips it of its nutrients. Because of this, table salt is much more damaging than white flour. Table salt should not be eaten by anyone, ever.

- Salt is vital to your well-being. Every culture that Weston A. Price studied had salt in their diets. Salt is critical for protein digestion, enzyme activation of carbohydrates, and development of the brain and adrenal glands. The adrenal cortex, or outer layer of the adrenal glands, has a large need for salt. In today's fast-paced society, it's no wonder that so many people crave salt. A high-quality salt is full of as many as eighty important minerals your body needs, and it doesn't accelerate blood pressure problems as does table salt. In addition, high- quality salt is vital for balancing blood sugar levels, energy production, the proper absorption of nutrients, maintaining a proper pH, nerve-cell communication, and information processing,

- Salt, in combination with water, regulates the flow of water and wastes between the inside and the outside of your cells. During a cleansing plan such as this, it is essential to have a healthy source of salt. When you use sea salt, you don't have to limit your intake of salt in the same way that you must limit the use of table salt. If you happen to love salt on your food, this is good news! And for those of you who have limited your salt consumption, please do start enjoying salt with your meals.

Processed, Smoked, or Commercial Meats Including Farm-Raised Fish

Essential Guideline:
One of the most important ingredients to avoid in this category is MSG. Celtic sea salt is a healthy ingredient and may be consumed liberally.

Additional Details:

- These meats also are full of synthetic chemicals that weaken our bodies.

- Animals raised for commercial meat production live in environments that cause the animal's body to be toxic, with the result that when we eat these meats, our body becomes more toxic. A toxic body requires more nutrients to handle the toxicity, and the demand for extra nutrients causes cellular malnutrition. It is important to realize that all diseases have at their root toxicity and cellular malnutrition.

FYI: A scoby is a pancake-shaped kombucha culture (Note: scoby is an acronym for symbiotic culture of bacteria and yeast).

Never store your scoby in the refrigerator or put it in the freezer. Scobies are alive and may be stored in kombucha tea at room termperature.

FYI: Coconut oil raises body temperature, boosts metabolism, and gives you energy. These characteristics are often helpful for people who have low thyroid.

FYI: Butter, eggs, and coconut oil help suppress sugar cravings.

CHAPTER SIX

Five-Day Nutritious-Liquids Fast

"So much of our truly meaningful cultural events were at one time based upon food; the harvest, the feast, fasting or restricted eating, disciplined religious food choices. Modern society has been cut loose from these anchors that were so important to our ancestors, the knowledge ceased to be passed down when we gave up our responsibility to feed ourselves to big business. If we take back that responsibility we can usher in a rebirth of the community spirit that is so lacking today."

-Nel Stemm

I strongly advise that you do not partake of a fast without preparing, especially if you are already ill. I have seen too many people come out of a fast with a new set of chronic symptoms. The amount of stored-up toxins that can be released into the blood stream can do serious damage not only to your liver, but also to your entire body. Due to the high amount of toxins that we are exposed to today, fasting is best preceded by a cleansing diet. Please consult your physician before you begin a fast.

Fasting has been a powerful healing tool for many peoples for many years, but as we have read, fasting must be integrated with other elements of a good life. Few people realize just how many toxins are stored in each and every one of our cells due to our modern lifestyles. Toxic chemicals pose an elevated cancer risk to two-thirds of Americans living in nearly every part of the United States. Even the United States Environmental Protection Agency, whose standards are much lower than they need to be, has stated that toxic chemicals threaten each and every person in this country. It is also known that plastic by-products can be detected in the blood of EVERY human on the planet, and these do not degrade, nor does the body have the ability to get rid of these without proper nutrients and treatment.

A Fasting Experience That Will Change the Way You Feel

Because many people have lost the art of living well and because there are so many toxins in our environment, most people equate misery with the idea of fasting. For my clients, this is not the case. When you prepare for a fast, as you have with the OHC Plan, you realize that a fast can be rejuvenating and even thrilling. The fasting experience laid out in this book can change the way you feel about your body, your power to choose what you eat, and your ability to tell how different foods make you feel. After a fast, YOU CAN TELL THAT YOU FEEL HEALTHIER. Feeling healthier makes you want to keep feeling healthier. Often, after this five-day liquid diet, you feel so much healthier that you commit to always eating well.

The Joy of Fasting

Every client I work with that follows this 35-day plan is always amazed at how great they feel, how stable their blood sugar is and how much energy they have during the fasting process. Here's why:

- They have prepared their body for the fasting process

- They are cleaning out their colon

- They are ingesting an assortment of nutritious supplements that are assisting their body with detoxification

- They are eating raw fats and proteins and not starving their body

- They are drinking one-half gallon to one-whole gallon of nutritious liquids in addition to their daily water intake

In total, this is an easy fast that will lead to better health.

Resting and Healing

Fasting programs actually let your body concentrate on resting and healing, since the daily energy drain needed to complete the digestion cycle is reduced. Your bodily organs get a chance to rest and rebuild their functions while your white blood cells work at destroying up to 50 percent more unhealthy microorganisms. Plus, your body is able to slough off virulent cells and old accumulations of toxins. Fasting is your body's way to get rid of unwanted elements and to help the recovery process. A fine example of the power of fasting is that when we are sick with the flu, your body demands that you don't eat in order to heal.

During this fast, you will need to take in not only your regular amounts of water, but you will also need to consume nutritious liquids. If we evoke our cultural and medical tradition of fasting, we can clearly see that by using raw milk during fasting you have a combination of a detoxifying fast and a nutrient-dense feeding.

Nutritious Liquids are the Key to a Successful Fast

Nutritious liquids will keep your blood sugar balanced and they can be taken freely throughout the day to feel full and prevent you from feeling hungry. In order to keep your blood sugar stable and to help your body discard toxins, you'll need to drink liquids that contain fat and protein. Examples include:

- Raw milk
- Soup broth made from bones with options such as raw eggs and coconut oil

These easy-to-digest liquids may be combined with small amounts of nutritious liquids that contain carbohydrates. Examples include:

- Carrot juice
- Fruit juice
- Beet kvass
- Kombucha

FYI: Soy protein is promoted to upscale, health-conscious shoppers. In her book, *The Whole Soy Story*, author Kaayla Daniel explains how soy causes health problems in adults and children.

FYI: Most people do not realize that our bodies are always cleansing. Enemas are an extremely safe, effective and economical way to assist the body with this process.

Worried About Hunger During Your Fast?

If you're worried about hunger during your fast, prepare plenty of bone broth and add raw egg or coconut milk to increase the fat content (Note: try these recipes ahead of time to determine how much of these liquids you'd like to include during your fast). Organic coconut milk is available in cans and it's a delicious addition to chicken broth. Don't buy the Lite version because you'll want the fat content. The following recipes will make your broth interesting and you may want to add root vegetables to these soups at a later date:

Coconut Chicken Broth

Note: This is a variation of Sally Fallon's Easy Coconut Chicken Soup made without the solid ingredients.

1 can coconut milk
1 quart chicken stock
1-inch piece grated ginger
1 teaspoon sea salt
Juice of 1 lemon or 2 limes
1 tablespoon fresh basil leaves

Place the ingredients in a sauce pan and bring to a boil. Reduce the heat and simmer for 30 minutes.

Egg Drop Soup

My egg drop soup has a thinner texture than traditional Chinese egg drop soup because I do not use corn starch to thicken the broth. Although you've seen my warnings about soy throughout the book, soy sauce is fermented and can be used in recipes in small quantities.

1 quart chicken stock
1-inch piece grated ginger
3 eggs, beaten
1 tablespoon of soy sauce

Place all the ingredients except the eggs in a sauce pan and bring to a boil. Reduce the heat to a simmer and pour the egg mixture through a strainer while stirring the soup. The egg will coagulate and form delicate feathers in your broth.

Planning Your Fast

Two to three weeks before your fast, you'll want to start determining which nutritious liquid are right for you. Here are some suggestions:

- By this time, you have most likely determined whether or you not you can access raw milk. If you can, drink as much raw milk on this fast as you wish. Remember that the realmilk. com Web site lists sources of raw milk in each state. In addition, the Optimal Health Center can help you find raw milk sources that may not be listed in resource directories. (Note: If you feel bloated or gassy after drinking raw milk, try raw cheese and raw butter instead. If your body is sensitive to these products, raw dairy may not be for you).

  Note: Try hard to find a source of raw milk. If you absolutely cannot buy raw milk in your area, you will need to rely on the bone broth recipes and experiment with a raw egg or coconut milk for added fat.

- Make bone broth using the recipe in this book. I like to make bone broth in a five or six quart stock pot through the night. In the morning, I strain the broth into a large bowl and place it in the refrigerator for a day or two. I skim off the thick layer of fat that forms on the top of the broth and then I fill quart-sized Mason jars leaving an inch of space at the top. These jars may either be stored in the refrigerator or placed in the freezer. If you make broth with a whole chicken or chicken pieces, freeze the meat for future recipes.

- Make vegetable juice and experiment with vegetable juice combinations to determine the juices that you like.

FYI: Hair Mineral Analysis (HTMA) is a helpful way to identify heavy metal toxins that may be present in your body. In order to fully remove heavy metals from your body, you will need to do more than this 35-day program. Possible options include:

- Herbs such a cilantro and China Chlorella are natural chelators.

- Magnetic clay baths available from www. optimalhealthnetwork. com. If metal toxins are unknown, the Clear-Out formula is a general formula that removes lead, arsenic, mercury and aluminum.

Finding Non-Toxic Pots, Pans and Food Containers

Many of my readers are already familiar with the topic of safe pots and pans. Here's a review of the non-toxic options:

Glass

Glass pans are considered to be one of the healthiest options. Although there are white glass casserole dishes sold in the national chain stores, glass sauce pans have been discontinued. Howver, you can still find them at thrift stores and on eBay.

Porcelain

Porcelain covered aluminum is considered safe as long as there are no chips or cracks. These pans are light weight and very reasonably priced. For example, Martha Stewart has a line of light-weight gray-colored porcelain pots that are sold at K-Mart.

Teflon

Teflon scratches easily and it toxic at very high temperatures. If you're careful with your pans, teflon is an acceptable option that's safe to use for short, stove-top cooking.

Cast Iron

Cast iron was once considered to be one of the healthiest options. However, Raymond Peat, a respected naturopath in Eugene, Oregon, has explained that excess iron is very toxic. In a newlsetter article called "Iron's Dangers" he writes:

"Just like lead, mercury, cadmium, nickel and other heavy metals, stored iron produces destructive free radicals. The harmful effects of iton-produced free radicals are practically indistinguishable from those causes by exposure to X-rays and gamma rays; both accelerate the accumulation of age-pigment and other signs of aging."

Stainless Steel

Raymond Peat explains that there are two main types of stainless steel, magnetic and nonmagnetic. The nonmagnetic form has a very high nickel content. He explains that nickel is much more toxic than iron or aluminum. It's both allergenic and carcinogenic. To test for safe stainless, use a refrigerator magnet to determine which pans contain a high amount of nickel. The magnet will stick to the safer type of pan.

FYI: Cruciferous vegetables such as broccoli, cabbage and brussel sprouts depress the thyroid. Cooking or fermenting neutralizes thyroid-suppressing compounds in these vegetables.

- Make kombucha and/or beet kvass to see if these drinks are for you.

- Purchase organic gourmet broths or purees at your local health food store to see if you like these liquids.

Shopping and Planning

Once you've made your sample liquids and selected your choices for your fast, the next step is to purchase and prepare enough for your fast (*Note: See my shopping list near the end of this chapter*).

You'll need a minimum of two-to-four quarts of some protein liquid and one pint-to one quart of carbohydrate liquid for each day of your fast. Some people like to consume only protein liquids during a fast. There's no limit on the amount of liquid you're allowed to consume. Keep in mind that the liquids that contain protein and fat will keep you satisfied and they'll help you keep your blood sugar levels stable. The carbohydrate liquids are optional and they should only be consumed in small quantities.

If you do not take time off from work during your fast, you'll need to take two-to-three 15-ounce thermos containers with you to work. Although the newer thermos containers have larger capacities, they're lined with stainless steel that does not pass the refrigerator magnet safety test described in the next section. If your stainless steel thermos bottle passes the refrigerator magnet safety test and can hold more than 15 ounces, by all means use it! The older thermos bottles lines with glass are the safest option and they're available at www.thermos.com.

Raw Milk

Essential Guideline:

Raw milk is your most important food during your fast. You may drink raw goat's milk, raw cow's milk, or raw organic coconut milk.

Additional Details:

- Many people will not know where (or how) to buy raw milk.

- To find a local source of raw cow's milk, go to www.realmilk.com. Coconut milk may be found in ethnic food stores, at natural food stores and at www.wildernessfamilynaturals.com.

Living Fuel

Essential Guideline:

Living Fuel is an optimized super-food meal replacement.

Additional Details:

- Living Fuel contains many nutrients, and is designed to be hypoallergenic and to have a low glycemic response. It is a blend of potent, organic, wildcrafted, and natural foods that have been optimized with bio-available and usable nutrients and co-factor, including stabilized probiotics for healthy intestinal functioning.

- Living Fuel also contains herbs to enhance major body systems; antioxidants to protect against free-radical damage; vitamins and minerals to optimize the naturally occurring vitamin and mineral profiles of the foods; amino acids to optimize the naturally occurring amino acid profile of the plant proteins; and a custom enzyme complex to maximize the delivery of nutrients to the body which provides complete building blocks and fuel for the body, brain, and every cell in a nutrient-dense restricted carbohydrate format. It's easy.

Fresh Vegetable Juices

Essential Guideline:
Vegetables include celery, cucumber, and greens, with a little carrot, lemon, or beet added for flavor.

Additional Details:

- Muir Glen Vegetable Juice is an acceptable brand that may be used.

- Vegetables—lightly steamed or raw and blended or mixed in the Vita mix is an optional way to prepare vegetable juice for your liquid fast. You may add soup broth.

- A "Blended Salad" is also included in this category:

  Ingredients:
  1 medium tomato
  3 in. piece of cucumber, unpeeled, or peeled if waxed
  1 small red or green bell pepper, seeds removed
  2 cups lettuce pieces
  1 large celery stalk
  1 avocado

  Directions: Liquefy the tomato and cucumber in a blender or Vita Mix. Add pepper, avocado, and lettuce, using the celery stalk to push leaves down while the mixer runs on medium. Liquefy celery. Add water to preferred consistency.

Soups

Essential Guideline:
This category includes a few easy-to-prepare vegetable soups as well as bone broths made from poultry.

Additional Details:

- Chicken or Turkey broth

  Note: Turkey parts may be substituted for chicken parts in this recipe.

FYI: Lee Dexter, who owns White Egret Farms in Austin, Texas, studied the government data on the Centers for Disease Control (CDC) Web site and found that raw milk is the safest food in our food supply. It is:

- 2.5 times safer than pasterurized
- 3.5 times safer than other foods (for details, see www.realmilk.org)

Ingredients:
1 whole free-range chicken or chicken parts
4 quarts filtered water
2 tablespoons vinegar
1 large onion, chopped
2 carrots, peeled and chopped
3 celery sticks, chopped
1 bunch parsley

Directions: Place the chicken or chicken parts into a large stainless steel pot with water, vinegar and all vegetables except parsley. Let the pot stand for 30-to-60 minutes. Bring to a boil, and remove the scum from the surface. Reduce the heat and simmer for 6-to-24 hours. Add parsley about 10 minutes before the stock is finished. Remove the chicken from the broth and use the meat for other recipes. Strain the broth into a large bowl and place this liquid into your refrigerator until the fat congeals on the surface. Skim off the fat and store the broth in glass containers in your refrigerator or freezer.

- Quick Soup

Ingredients:
1 head broccoli or any vegetable (2-3 cups) steamed
Favorite spices
1 cup water
½ to 1 cup raw dairy to desired consistency

Directions: Steam vegetables until very soft. Take vegetables and water from steamer and pour into blender or Vita mix. Add ½ cup raw milk and blend on high until liquefied. If too thick, add more raw dairy. Add sea salt and/or spices if desired.

Herbal Teas

Essential Guideline:
Herbal tea (1 cup only per day) or water with Glycerine (1 tablespoon per qt.)

Additional Details:

- Healthy herbal tea choices include nettle, peppermint, and Pau d' Arco. Regular tea contains fluoride. Scientists believe that fluoride is absorbed naturally into tea plants from soil and rainwater.

- Glycerine is a healthy sweetener made out of coconuts.

Beet Kvass

Essential Guideline:
This lacto-fermented drink is valuable for its medicinal qualities and as a digestive aid. Beets are just loaded with nutrients.

Additional Details:

- One 4-oz. glass, morning and night, is an excellent blood tonic, promotes regularity, aids digestion, alkalizes the blood, cleanses the liver, and is a good treatment for kidney stones and other ailments. After the fast, beet kvass may also be used in place of vinegar in salad dressing and as an addition to soups.

- Ingredients:
  3 medium or 2 large organic beets
  peeled and chopped up coarsely
  ¼ cup whey
  1 tablespoon Celtic Sea Salt
  filtered water

- Directions: Makes 2 quarts.
  Place beets, whey, and salt in a 2-quart glass container. Add filtered water to fill the container. Stir well and cover securely. Keep at room temperature for 2 days before transferring to refrigerator.

  When most of the liquid has been drunk, you may fill up the container with water and keep it at room temperature another 2 days. The resulting brew will be slightly less strong than the first. After the second brew, discard the beets and start again. You may, however, reserve some of the liquid and use this as your innoculant instead of the whey.

FYI: Sally Fallon explains that our ancestors had one of the healthiest diets on the planet that included pasture-based agriculture and a lot of butter.

Note: Do not use grated beets in the preparation of beet tonic. When grated, beets exude too much juice which results in a too-rapid fermentation that favors the production of alcohol rather than lactic acid.

Kefir

Essential Guideline:

Kefir is a yogurt-like lacto-fermented beverage with a slightly fizzy taste that is made from kefir grains. It has thirty times more probiotic cultures than yogurt, including lactobacillus acidophilus and bifidobacteria.

Additional Details:

- Kefir's live yeast and bacteria cultures can colonize the intestinal tract to control and eliminate destructive pathogenic microorganisms. When this happens, the body becomes more efficient in resisting such pathogens as E. coli and intestinal parasites.

- Ingredients/equipment:
  Glass Jar with a plastic lid (look for marshmallow or mayonnaise jars that are glass with plastic lids).
  3-quart plastic strainer with small holes
  Wooden spoon or plastic spatula
  Kefir grains

- Directions: The kefir-making e-group at Yahoo has over 3,000 members (http://groups.yahoo.com/group/Kefir_making). The people who post regularly will help you find kefir grains. If grains need to be mailed, they will survive in a double-Ziploc baggie with a small amount of milk for two-to-three days. The Yahoo group members usually do not expect payment but they will need to be reimbursed for postage.

- When your grains arrive, immediately transfer them to a glass jar and add one cup of milk (Note: the milk can be cold). The lid should be loosely fitted. Place the jar on a shelf or your counter at room temperature. Swirl the jar at five second intervals whenever possible.

- Approximately 24 hours after you have started your kefir, your product will be very thick. It may start to separate into curds and whey.

- As the grains multiply, fermentation will accelerate. You'll want to strain your kefir when you see a separation beginning to take place.

- Use the spatula or wooden spoon to push your grains into a clean jar to start a new batch. Do not place grains into a jar that is warm from a dishwasher.

- Swirling breaks up the grains and exposes more surfaces to lactose.

- Grains multiply at a rate of 10 percent per day in the summer and 5 percent per day in the winter.

- Use an empty milk carton to store finished kefir in the refrigerator.

- Grains may be covered with milk and placed in the refrigerator to hibernate. Change the milk at least once-a-week and don't let the grains hibernate for a prolonged period of time.

- There are three ways to slow down your kefir:

  1. Add more milk

  2. Remove some of your grains (Note: you can eat the grains or give them away to a friend)

Kombucha

Essential Guideline:
This fizzy lacto-fermented beverage is a natural soft drink that is most known for it's vitamin B, Folic Acid, and glucoronic acid content.

FYI: In a perky report called "Mooing recyclers" that was published in the April 26, 2005 issue of Madison, Wisconsin's *Capitol Times*, writer Caroline Peterson described the waste from food manufactuing that's fed to Wisconsin's dairy cows. She wrote:

"Instead of the usual mundane meal of dry hay, chopped silage, and ground corn, many of Wisconsin's dairy cows munch on over-cooked potato chips, mangled gummy bears, and discarded chocolate balls along with their fodder."

Fortunately, there's a growing organic movement in Wisconsin that consists of dairy farmers who feed their cows healthy grass and not waste products.

Additional Details:

- Glucoronic acid is a conjugate that moves toxins out of the body.

- Vitamins B6, B12, and Folic Acid prevent a wide range of neurologic and cardiovascular conditions including, Alzheimer's Disease, Parkinson's Disease, schizophrenia, multiple sclerosis, cognitive decline, and heart disease. Although fermented vegetables do not contain the same form of Vitamin B12 that is found in meat, milk and eggs, studies show that B6, B12 and Folic acid work alone as well as synergistically.

- Equipment
  Tea kettle (stainless steel or porcelain enamel).

  Steeping container (appropriate Pyrex container).

  Glass brewing container (gallon-size cookie jar offers a wide mouth for maximum air exposure and easy cleaning).

  Cotton cover (piece of tightly woven cotton will be needed to cover the brew with a strong rubber band. Kitchen towels and cotton dinner napkins may be cut up for this purpose).

  Wooden spoon, plastic spatula (nonmetal utensil will be needed to remove the tea bags from your brew).

  Glass or plastic measuring cup (medium or large-size measuring cup will be needed to measure water and sugar).

  Cheesecloth (provides a fine mesh to strain your kombucha).

  Plastic funnel (optional: helpful for bottling your brew, and you can also use the lip on your measuring cup to pour the liquid).

  Glass straining container (a second gallon-size cookie jar or a 64 oz. Pyrex is a useful straining container).

  Bottles (glass is suitable for bottling. It is important that the bottle does not have a metal cap. At room temperature, gas will accumulate in a closed container. If you leave your kombucha out of the refrigerator and you don't drink it right away, you will need to release the accumulated gas. Always open kombucha bottles carefully in case there is a gas build-up).

- Ingredients
  Black and Green Tea (six tea bags, 3 black and 3 green; use tea bags that do not have staples. Tetley black and Celestial Seasonings green do not have staples).

  1 cup refined white sugar (organic white granulated sugar may be used, brown sugar makes an inferior brew).

  3 quarts of filtered water.

  SCOBY: a pancake-shaped kombucha culture (SCOBY is an acronym for symbiotic culture of bacteria and yeast).

  Starter liquid: a strong (acidic) liquid from the mother's brew.

  White vinegar: Many people use white vinegar for cleaning and rinsing. White vinegar is not made with a culture and will not contaminate a brew.

- Directions: The original kombucha e-group at Yahoo has members willing to share their scobies (http://groups.yahoo.com/group/original_kombucha). If a scoby needs to be mailed, it will survive in a double-Ziploc baggie with a small amount of kombucha for four to five days. Yahoo group members usually do not expect payment but they will need to be reimbursed for postage.

- Boil one quart of water and place the water in a suitable steeping container with the six tea bags and one cup sugar. The sugar will dissolve immediately.

- Steep your tea concentrate for a minimum of 15 minutes. Remove the tea bags with a nonmetal utensil when the liquid is sufficiently cooled.

- Add two quarts of water to your brewing container.

- Add the concentrate to the clear water in your brewing container. Allow the liquid to completely cool to room temperature.

FYI: Processed foods contain not only dangerous neurotoxins, but also trans-fats that are spoiled vegetables oils that have been heated to very high temperatures and then processed to preserve shelf life.

- Remove your jewelry, rinse your hands with white vinegar, and place your SCOBY in the brewing container with the "top" side up (look for "top-side" on the bag it came in). Slowly pour one cup of starter liquid (provided with your SCOBY) on top. This acidic liquid (brew for 12 days) helps prevent mold from forming. Some SCOBIES float and others sink. In either case, a baby will grow on the top of the liquid.

- Attach your cotton cover to the jar with a rubber band and place your brew in a quiet, semidark area where it won't be disturbed (Note: 73-80 degrees is best). The cotton cover will protect your brew from fruit flies.

Days	Kombucha
7-8	Sweet and fizzy
9	Slightly tart
12-23	Acidic (Starter liquid)

- On the day you would like to strain your kombucha, remove your jewelry, rinse your hands with white vinegar and carefully remove your SCOBY (mother and newly formed baby) from the brewing container and place the pair on a clean plate.

- Cut a square of cheesecloth to cover a straining container. Secure the cheesecloth with a rubber band.

- Pour all of the brew through the cheese cloth. The loose weave will allow healthy particles into your kombucha. The brown sediment is yeast.

- Pour most of the brew into bottles (reserve at least 2 cups to store your SCOBIES—one cup for the mother and one cup for the baby). Fill the bottles completely to the top to limit any air. Leave the bottles out at room temperature for four to five days (for a fizzier brew) or place them in the refrigerator.

- Leave a minimum of 2 cups of liquid in the bottom of your alternate brewing jar to store your scoby until day 12. The extra days will make an acidic starter for you to use with the mother and baby in your next brew. Place the SCOBIES (mother and baby) back in the quiet place where the kombucha has been brewing.

FYI: Raw milk has been sold legally in California for many years without problems.

- Remove your jewelry, rinse your hands with white vinegar, and carefully remove your scoby (mother and baby) from the brewing container and place the pair on a clean plate.

Shopping Guide
This simple shopping list is provided as a review to help you prepare for your fast.

Review: Products You'll Need

1. Vit-Ra-Tox Kit
Purchase this kit from www.optimalhealthnetwork.com.

2. Quality Water
If you're drinking quality water, you will need to research this topic (See: Chapter 4) .

3. Nutritious Liquids
Most people will need to pick two or three liquids from this list due to the ease-of-access or ease-of-preparation or both. If you have access to all of the nutritious liquids and you feel comfortable using all of them, feel free to create a liquid fast diet using all of the liquids. You will need to drink 1/2 to 1 gallon of nutritious liquids each day and having a couple of thermoses on hand allows you to travel with your liquids.

- Raw Milk
- Living Fuel
- Fresh, organic vegetable juice
- Home-made bone broth or packaged soup
- Beet Kvass
- Kefir
- Kombucha

---

4. Coconut Oil

Coconut oil will keep you warm, cleanse your liver and help your body remove toxins. It will also help you feel full and reset your metabolism while you fast. Take two to three tablespoons of coconut oil each day. Sally Fallon and her co-author Mary Enig have written extensively about the health benefits of coconut oil in their book *Eat Fat, Lose Fat*. Coconut oil is available at www.optimalhealthnetwork.com.

Additional Details

1. Raw Milk

If you're having trouble locating raw milk, contact your nearest Weston A. Price chapter. Check the following list on the Web: www.westonaprice.org/localchapters/locallist.html.

2. Very Veggie

Very Veggie is a delicious, tomato-based, organic vegetable juice. To locate a supplier, check: www.knudsenjuices.com.

3. Bone Broth

The chicken or turkey bones in the stock recipe can be replaced with any other meat bones such as lamb, beef, buffalo, fish or venison. For additional stock recipes, refer to Sally Fallon's Nourishing Traditions cookbook.

4. Organic Gourmet Broth

Imagine Foods and Pacific Foods make delicious, organic gourmet broth. These broths are made from orrganically-raised free-range chickens, organic beef and organic vegetables. If you cannot make your own broth, look for single-serving and family-sized packages from these companies (See: www.imaginefoods.com and www.pacificfoods.com).

5. Teas

Hot chamomile tea with raw cream is a treat at bedtime. Peppermint tea in the mid-afternoon also brings a sense of digestive health during a fast. My other favorite teas include Echinacea, Nettle Leaf, Pau D'Arco and Oat Straw. I recommend one-to-four cups of herbal tea daily.

Eliminating Toxins From Your Body

During a fast, what you remove from your body is just as important as what you put into your body. Most people need to eliminate more waste and toxins than they can naturally eliminate on a daily basis. It is essential during a fast to remove from your colon at least 20 feet of stool. Twenty feet is what you ought to remove when you fast for five days. On a longer fast, you would want to remove more than twenty feet. Without colon cleansing, the toxins released as a result of the fast can actually be re-absorbed into your bloodstream because you are not eliminating the requisite 2 to 20 feet of stool daily through your colon. This happens due to the fact that one of the main jobs of the colon is to absorb liquids. When the body re-absorbs your hard-earned toxic waste, you are much more likely to experience pain and the illnesses typically associated with a cleansing fast. Colon cleansing is going to be very helpful and crucial during your fast because it is helping to prevent the re-absorption of toxins. This is why I always recommend that people take at least three days worth of therapeutic enemas or have colon hydrotherapy performed on three different days during the five-day fast, as a minimum amount of colon cleansing.

The "Ropes" Called Mucoid Plaque

During the colonic, or enema process, you will see some unusual excrement coming from your body. This is no cause for concern. These "ropes" are called *mucoid plaque*. They are a mixture of the psyllium fiber and bentonite clay from the Vit-Ra-Tox kit used during the deep tissue cleanse. They are loaded with the many toxins that are being cleared from every part of the body. I do not think that these "ropes" actually line the walls of the colon, but rather, are formed as the toxins, bacterial waste, bile, fiber and clay combine while moving through the colon. Again, when using the OHC Plan cleanse, my clients actually move 2 to 20 feet of these "ropes" out of their colon per day.

The Importance of Supplements

It is essential during your fast that you take supplements. Without them, you will not remove as many of the toxins that are being released as you need to do for a successful cleanse. I recommend

FYI: The Weston A. Price Foundation is seeing many cases of children who are dying before their parents.

V.E. Irons' Vit-Ra-Tox kit. The fiber in the Vit-Ra-Tox kit will give the toxins, bacterial waste and debris, which are leaving your body, something to adhere to while passing through your colon. The clay carries a negative electric charge and can attract positively charged pathogenic organisms along with their toxins and carry them out of the body. Clay compounds also provide minerals. As such, bentonite clay facilitates assimilation of the nutrients you are taking in from raw milk and vegetable juices and can help the intestines to rid the body of toxins that are being released from cells.

The other supplements in the Vit-Ra-Tox kit are Greenlife , a combination of grasses, vitamin C, and Wheat Germ/Flax oil. These will bring into your body the extra nutrients needed to keep your immune system fully functional while you do the hard work of fasting. I have worked with many other similar products, but the Vit-Ra-Tox kit always brings about the most consistent results with components that are safe and of the highest quality.

Five-Day Fasting Calendar

When you schedule your fast, consider giving yourself a little extra time everyday to process your cleansing experience, and possibly even squeeze in a nap. You might pick a week or a long weekend to start the plan. Healing takes energy. On the other hand, with good planning, this regimen easily fits into most people's busy schedule's. Most people I work with apply this plan within their busy schedules.

Day/Fast	Component
1	Nutritious Liquids
	Vit-Ra-Tox kit
	Supplements
	Therapeutic Enema
2	Nutritious Liquids
	Vit-Ra-Tox kit
	Supplements
	Hydrotherapy Session (or Therapeutic Enema)

3	Nutritious Liquids
	Vit-Ra-Tox kit
	Supplements
	Hydrotherapy Session (or Therapeutic Enema)
4	Nutritious Liquids
	Vit-Ra-Tox kit
	Supplements
	Therapeutic Enema
5	Nutritious Liquids
	Vit-Ra-Tox kit
	Supplements
	Hydrotherapy Session (or Therapeutic Enema)

Daily/Hourly Schedule for the Five-Day Nutritious Liquids Fast

Upon rising, start taking your psyllium and bentonite from your supplement kit. You will take 1 level tablespoon of bentonite and 1 heaping teaspoon of psyllium. Along with this, drink at least ten ounces of water. You will repeatedly take the psyllium and bentonite for a total of four times throughout the day (five times if you weigh over 150 pounds).

Roughly one-and-one-half hours after taking the psyllium and bentonite, take the tablet supplements. I recommend that you take eight Greenlife, two Wheat Germ/Flax Oil tablets, and two vitamin C pills. These will also be taken for a total of four to five times each day.

Time	Component
7:00 a.m.	Water/psyllium/bentonite
8:30 a.m.	Water and tablets
10:00 a.m.	Water/psyllium/bentonite
11:30 a.m.	Water and tablets
1:00 p.m.	Water/psyllium/bentonite

FYI: The September 2004 issue of the *Danish Research Centre for Organic Farming* newsletter reported a higher antioxidant content in organic milk than in conventional milk due to feeding strategy. The higher concentrations of vitamin E and carotenoids in organic milk are a result of feeding differences between the conventional and the organic production methods. The most important reason for the observed differences is presumably the large amounts of maize silage used in conventional production, whereas a considerable amount of grass and leguminous plants are used in organic production.

FYI: In 2003, Public Citizen sponsored a "Factory Farm" tour for nine farmers from around the world, in an effort to connect people who are working to stop inhumane, environmentally damaging factory farming.

Traveling by bus, they visited large hog and dairy operations, as well as family farms, in Iowa and Wisconsin.

A new video, "Through Farmers Eyes: The Impacts of Industrialized Agriculture," documents their travels through the Midwest and their reactions to the industrial model of farming that is starting to invade their own countries.

If you would like to receive a complimentary copy of the 22-minute documentary, please e-mail cmep@citizen.org. Please specify DVD or VHS in your e-mail.

2:30 p.m.	Water and tablets
4:00 p.m.	Water/psyllium/bentonite
5:30 p.m.	Water and tablets

(For those who weigh over 150 pounds):

7:00 p.m.	Water/psyllium/bentonite
8:30 p.m.	Water and tablets

Helpful Hints

If you get off schedule, just start again. Using a watch with a timer can help tremendously during these five days. The main goal here is to get the correct amount into your body, at equally spaced intervals, over the course of a day. Dividing up the dosages and placing them in small containers can help you to stay on track during your busy day, even outside of the house. Make sure you don't premix the psyllium with a liquid, as it will turn into cement. You can add the bentonite to water for easy carrying. Also, a day's worth of tablets fit nicely into a pillbox or plastic baggie.

The Day After: Breaking Your Fast

It can be said that the most important aspect of a fast is how you end it. The worst thing you can do is give your digestive tract a great cleanse and then eat a large amount of hard-to-digest foods! Even if you've been thinking about stuffed pizza all week–don't do it! You could hurt your stomach and small intestines and feel awful afterwards.

If you've been having cravings throughout the cleanse and are now tempted to satisfy them, keep thinking clearly. It is important to be aware that your cravings may be caused by the ongoing discharging of toxins. Take your therapeutic enemas. Also, the cravings could be caused by emotional work that has come to your awareness because of the fast. Grab a friend and tell your life story. Cry hard. Laugh uncontrollably. Find yourself a space where you can do the healing work that is being brought up for you. If you need more support for the emotional work you face, you may find the tools of co-counseling extremely helpful. For more information, go to www.rc.org.

When ending your nutritious-liquids fast, always start eating by adding very small amounts of easy-to-digest food. Going back to how you ate on your OHC plan, at least for a couple of days, is a very wise idea. After these few days, if you are going to add in foods that aren't on the OHC plan, please add them in one at a time. In other words, give your body a chance to let you know if some food is particularly hard on it by adding in foods one at a time. Besides, my goal for you is that you will follow the OHC plan for the rest of your life.

FYI: Mark Purdy is an organic dairy farmer from Somerset, England, who refused to obey British government orders to spray his cattle with organophosphates—a chemical— in order to fight the warble fly. Purdy went to court to challenge the order and won. His farm was exempted from using the spray. When the "Mad Cow" epidemic hit England, not one cow in Purdy's herd developed the disease. Purdy has studied the issue and argues that Mad Cow is not caused by a virus, but is a result of organo phosphate pesticides and toxic mineral overload.

-americanfreepress.net

FYI: The book-reviews section of the Weston A. Price Web site provides an in-depth analysis of famous diet books.

Notes

FYI: The Realmilk.org site created by the Weston A. Price Foundation contains a list of raw-milk sources in the United States and other countries. Lisitngs are arranged by state.

CHAPTER SEVEN

Colon Hydrotherapy

"The health of the colon is largely determined by the types of foods that are eaten. Equally as important as proper digestion is the proper elimination of waste products. A bowel movement every twelve to fourteen hours is critical to good health."

– Michael Murray, N. D

Colon hydrotherapy, colonics, and colon irrigation are an age-old health practice that gradually and soothingly cleanses the colon using water. During the administration of the colonic, a sanitary, FDA-approved system and disposable components are utilized. This state-of-the-art equipment has a fully integrated water-disinfecting system, a precision flow-control flow-meter, plus double safety components for trouble-free operation and peace of mind. The disinfecting system consists of a multistage water-filtration process that uses an ultraviolet sterilization process. Everything in this equipment is designed to provide a healthy, safe, cleansing process.

What to Expect

Once you and your therapist have discussed the procedure and you feel at ease with your new health venture, the two of you should establish your goals. Keeping these in mind, your therapist will typically advise you at this point of the schedule of colon cleansing that you will need to plan on in order to accomplish your goals. A series of colonics is generally required to bring the body back to a state of optimal health. Before starting the actual procedure, you are given a gown and asked to remove the appropriate clothing. Then you need to empty your bladder in the nearby toilet so your session won't be interrupted. After lying down on a comfortable padded table, a lubricated disposable speculum, having a tapered end, is gently inserted into the rectum. The tapered end is actually a separate piece that is removed after insertion and discarded. This is called an *obturator*. It is designed so that the insertion is not uncomfortable, nor is it damaging to any rectal tissue. The speculum is then attached to two tubes. The smaller tube delivers the filtered, temperature-controlled water to the speculum and your colon, while the larger tube carries the fecal waste to the colon therapy machine.

An 35-50 Minute Session

The closed system of colon therapy is attached to the building's plumbing system so that all waste is discreetly moved from your body into the plumbing without offensive odors or embarrassment. During your colonic sessions, your therapist will always make sure that your modesty and comfort needs are addressed. The machine has a viewing tube with special lighting that allows you to see (and the therapist to examine) what is coming out of your body. This provides you both an opportunity to discuss what is happening and for you to ask any questions regarding what you see. (I prefer and use in my clinic the "closed system" but there is also an "open system" that is equally as comfortable and effective).

During an average 35-50 minute session, a colon hydrotherapist infuses 30-50 gallons of filtered water into your body. At any one "fill," you may have between a pint and 2 quarts of water in your colon. During a fill, only the volume of water that feels comfortable for you is introduced. Once you feel full, you tell the therapist and the water is then released. Your colon empties out into the drainage tube carrying with it fecal and toxic matter that has been dislodged. This filling and emptying continues, along with abdominal massaging, for the entire session.

Cleansing Strengthens the Colon

This repetitive filling with water not only flushes waste out the colon, but it also stimulates the colon to contract. This contracting of the colon is called *peristalsis*. This is the same muscular action that the stool stimulates as it moves through the colon. In this way, colon cleansing with water is gentle and yet extremely effective, because as you clean the colon, you are strengthening the colonic musculature. This is why colon cleansing is not addictive, like laxatives, but is strengthening to your colon. Laxatives use chemicals to stimulate bowel movements, which is quite unnatural. Using water and essential oils to cleanse your colon can be an excellent way to bring about optimal bowel function.

Once you and your therapist feel you are done, you sit on the toilet for 5-15 minutes. Having a squatting stool available at the toilet can make a big difference, since a squatting stool allows the body to assume a position more conducive to comfortable expelling of colon waste. I recommend that clients really take their time while emptying on the toilet to bring about a full evacuation of the bowels as well as to increase their confidence that they won't have an accident on their way home.

Why Use Colon Hydrotherapy?
In order to answer this question, let's take a look at the colon's anatomy. The colon is what most people call their "gut" or their "stomach." When your "stomach" hurts, you are often really referring to your colon. Your colon is located in the lower abdomen, underneath your ribs and between your hips. It lies in this region like an upside-down U, or at least it ought to. The colon begins where the small intestine leaves off, at the cecum. It is about five feet long in adults.

The Colon's Main Structural Parts
The colon's main structural parts are called the *ascending, transverse*, *descending*, and *sigmoid* colon. The appendix is like a tail to the cecum. The ascending and transverse sections of the colon are the sites of re-absorption and secretion activities. Re-absorption of water and sodium dehydrates the colon content. The descending and sigmoid sections are sites of storage for fecal matter. The sigmoid joins the rectum, a muscular cavity with the ability to stimulate defecation. This all ends at the anus, which is the sphincter that keeps the stool in and lets the stool out when the musculature and nervous system determine that the lower colon is "full." In order to form solid stool, the ascending and transverse sections of the colon dehy-

FYI: Quality First is a company that has a patent on a centrifuge process for coconut oil. Although their products cannot be ordered online, details about their coconut oil may be found at:

qualityfirst.on.ca/

FYI: Jerry Brunetti is a well-known cancer survivor and advocate of Sally Fallon's *Nourishing Traditions*. His *Cancer, Nutrition & Healing* is available as a DVD on the Acres USA Web site: www.acresusa.com.

drate the materials (or the chyme) that have been delivered from the small intestines. (This is important to note in a discussion of colon cleansing, because the absorption of water during a treatment is another reason to be rigorous when choosing the quality of water you put into your colon.) Using the process of osmosis, the colon daily absorbs two to three quarts of water.

The Composition of Stool

As stool moves through the colon, it feeds the bacteria that produce many critical vitamins and digest cellulose and other fibers. In this way, as the content of your stool moves toward the rectum, the amount of solids with a dietary origin decreases, while the amount of solids with a bacterial origin increases.

This amazing design does its job well—for most of us. For others, there are problems. What is it about the colon in today's world that makes cleaning it such a great idea? There are many reasons, but let's take a look at just a few. Colon cancer is the second-leading cause of cancer death in the United States. Around 130,000 Americans are diagnosed with colon cancer annually. Doctors from one end of the country to the other are besieged with patients with digestive disorders like irritable bowel and these doctors have very little success in treating these conditions. Candida-related illnesses plague more people with confusing symptoms every day. Chemical sensitivities are common, whereas just ten years ago they were relatively unheard of. Each and every day, we ingest toxic chemicals that need to be removed before they are stored into our cells. Toxic chemicals lodged in our organs cause many chronic health problems All of these health problems, in one way or another, point to the fact that the colon needs help.

The Colon Needs Help

At this point you might ask, "Doesn't it clean itself? We don't clean any of our other internal body parts." Actually, we do! We clean our teeth and gums. Just as we brush to maintain the health of our teeth and gums, it is plain good sense to "brush" our colon. As with the mouth, our colon is harmed, often without our awareness, by our daily choices. We live on a planet that has us regularly creating and ingesting substances that, while passing through the colonic barrier, often damage it, causing Leaky Gut Syndrome. Thus we risk losing our good health. Preventing harmful bacteria and yeast, environmental toxins, and undigested food particles from circulating in our bodies is a key role that the colon plays in keeping us healthy. By using colon cleansing to "clean" the colon, you strengthen the integrity of your colon, just as brushing strengthens the integrity of your teeth and gums.

We Live in a Polluted World

We don't eat well, and even those who do "eat well" tend to eat more sugar and starch than is healthy. We tend to be dehydrated. We live in a polluted world and absorb that pollution into our bodies everyday. We, as a culture, overuse antibiotics. Many women are taking birth-control substances that increase the overload state of the colon. More and more people are on prescription medications that cause constipation. We tend to be undernourished. We are under a tremendous amount of stress in our fast-paced lives. All of these tendencies lead to a breakdown in colon health.

Diminish the Toxic Load in the Entire Body

As the colon struggles to do its job, so does the liver. In order to have a healthy liver, most of us need to help our bodies eliminate the incredible amount of waste and toxins that are in our bodies. Colon hydrotherapy plays a crucial role in this process, because when we cleanse the colon, we substantially diminish the toxic load in the entire body. With fewer toxins, the entire body experiences less stress and can devote more energy to healing and maintaining a healthy state.

One specific example of the benefits of colon cleansing can be examined by looking at the role the gallbladder plays in the body. The gallbladder, a digestive organ, stores bile, releasing it after meals for fat digestion. Bile also helps to carry out toxins that fat has become a carrier of. During a colon hydrotherapy session, there is often a tremendous release of bile. In this way, the body is helped to overcome toxicity, which is a common cause of many illnesses.

FYI: Sally Fallon has created a list of "Superfoods" at the back of her *Nourishing Traditions* cookbook. They're foods that concentrate important nutrients. Azomite Mineral Powder is on her list. It's a powder that's been mined from ancient sea beds in Utah for the last sixty years. Azomite is sold as a soil amendment but it's also valuable as a mineral supplement for animals and humans. A teaspoon mixed with water or some other liquid provides a source of silicon, calcium, magnesium and many trace minerals. Sally has told chapter leaders on her e-group that she takes it daily. For more information, see: www.azomite.com.

Due not only to our lifestyles, but also to our anatomy and physiology, the colon can often use our help. The entire anatomy of the digestive tract is built to be very selective about what it takes in and, especially, what it keeps out. For instance, the colon has unidirectional ileocecal valve, which connects the ileum of the small intestine with the cecum of the large intestine. One of the jobs of the ileocecal valve is to prevent bacteria of the colon from entering the normally clean small intestines and stomach. Millions of Americans suffer from gastric cancer, chronic abdominal pain, peptic ulcers, duodenal ulcers, and chronic gastritis. All of these ailments are scientifically connected to the presence of an overgrowth of the normally occurring Helicobacter pylori. When the colon is overloaded with stool and unhealthy bacteria and yeast, it struggles to do its job of keeping bacteria where it belongs. Colon cleansing can help.

The Colon's Job is More Important Than the Mouth's Job

The colon's job is more important than the mouth's job, and yet we expect it to optimally function on its own, without assistance. People ought to be moving at least one, if not two feet of stool, out of their bodies every single day of their lives. This stool should be at least the diameter of a US quarter, if not a US silver dollar. Obviously, there are many ways to make this happen, but for most of us, creating these ideal conditions in our day-to-day lives can be next to impossible. Yet, like brushing our teeth, colon cleansing becomes an excellent tool for keeping us healthy.

Frequently Asked Colon Hydrotherapy Questions

Over the years, many of my clients have asked a number of questions, including:

Question: *After colon hydrotherapy will I need to be close to the toilet all day?*

No, this is not a worry.

Question: *How will I feel during the session?*

Most people are nervous at first. After that, they relax. By the end of a session, generally people feel cleaner and healthier. As a therapist, I am also encouraged by the people who don't feel better after a session. A difficult colon therapy session can signal a distressed colon and progress being made to change that state.

Question: *Does it hurt?*

No. As your colon fills with water you may have some cramping. This is good. Your therapist uses this cue to empty your colon and assist you to release. Good communication with the therapist is what makes it a pain-free experience. I stay with the client during the entire treatment. This allows me to "work" the colon therapy machine in order to move out the 2-20 feet of stool during a regular session. Also, I pay attention to a person's body language as some people experience more discomfort than others. When someone is experiencing discomfort, I will massage their belly, or slow the flow of water, or let them sit on the toilet. One of the main jobs of the client is to tell me when they feel full. At this point, I will let the water that has been building up in the colon out. With the release of water comes stool.

Question: *Will I leak?*

No, most people don't leak. Part of the colon therapist's job is to diminish your chance of leaking by controlling the water flow and listening to you.

Question: *Will I make a mess all over?*
It is rare that a client makes a mess.

Question: *How long does it take?*
A colon hydrotherapy session usually takes between one-half hour to one hour.

Question: *How will I feel when I am finished?*

Some feel relaxed and a little tired, others feel empty or lighter, and 95% of my clients just feel great!

Question: *Is there any time I shouldn't have hydrotherapy?*

FYI: Dr. Raymond Peat, a respected naturopath in Eugene, Oregon, teaches his patients to use a refrigerator magnet when they shop for stainless steel pans. If the magnet sticks to a pan, it's a safe pan to buy. If the magnet does not stick, it means there's a lot of nickel content and nickel is toxic.

Yes. If you have uncontrolled hypertension or congestive heart failure, aneurysm, severe anemia, GI hemorrhage/perforation, severe hemorrhoids, renal insufficiency, cirrhosis, carcinoma of the colon, fistulas, abdominal hernia, recent colon surgery (less than three-months) or are in the first and third trimester of pregnancy, you shouldn't have hydrotherapy. If you have any of these conditions, using the OHC Plan without the colon therapy could reverse your symptoms.

Question: *Is colon hydrotherapy more effective than in-home enemas?*

Some people say yes, absolutely. Others only take enemas. In many ways, the effectiveness issue really comes down to personal preference and skill. You certainly do have access to a lot more water during a colon therapy session. Thirty to fifty gallons of water is more water than 6 quarts. Also, you have access to a trained professional with valuable experience. If you have access to colon hydrotherapy and you can afford it, I would definitely give it a try. In addition, this program can be very difficult to stick to at times. Setting up and paying for your colon therapy sessions at the start of your program can make all the difference in the world: You have made an agreement with another person and it is their job to support you in your process.

On the other hand, enemas are absolutely as effective as colon hydrotherapy. And, they are much cheaper. This gives you more money to spend on raw dairy, organics and other needed health tools. If you need help with taking enemas, read on and watch the videos, *All About Enemas*, and *Cleansing, Coffee Enemas, and Colon Tubes* at www.optimalhealthnetwork.com. These educational enema videos cover all you need to know about in-home enemas so that you can provide for yourself colon cleansing that has the same therapeutic value as a professional colon hydrotherapy session. I call these enemas therapeutic enemas.

Question: *I take daily fiber, shouldn't that do the trick?*

No, not necessarily. New studies show that fiber isn't necessarily the answer.

Question: *How often should I have colon therapy?*

Like brushing your teeth, you might choose to make colon cleansing a part of your regular hygiene program. Regular colon cleansing can be a very healthy choice.

There is no one prescription for all. A hair analysis gives you a picture of what toxins are stored in your body and what toxins you need to remove. Using the hair analysis on a seasonal basis will guide you to the cleansing program that will best suits your needs.

If you don't choose to utilize the hair analysis, know that most people find that after a colonic experience, they feel much better. It is this renewed vitality that is your guide. Keep it in mind. As soon as you find it diminishing, have a colon therapy session or a series of enemas. You'll find that in doing this you might feel better instantly. And, if you find that you don't feel better after a colon cleansing series, take a break for a period of time. In my clinic, it seems that most people benefit greatly from cleansing their colon at least one time per month.

FYI: Readers who wish to learn more about what takes place during a colon hyrdrotherapy session may wish to purchase a movie entitled *Using a Colonic to Cleanse Your Colon.* For further information, see: www.optimalhealthnetwork.com.

FYI: In 1913, Dr. Charles Sanford Porter wrote a book called *Milk Diet As a Remedy for Chronic Disease*. He believed that disease can only be cured by and through the blood—and that raw milk makes the purest and richest blood possible.

Notes

FYI: Over 3,000 people belong to the kefir-making e-group at Yahoo. A large number of the members reside in countries outside the United States.

CHAPTER EIGHT

Therapeutic Enemas

Enemas have been used for general purposes
of detoxification since ancient times.
-Charlotte Gerson and Morton Walker, D.P.M. The Gerson Therapy

A very long history of colon cleansing recommends enemas to improve immunity and to relieve ailments seemingly distinct from the digestive system.

For those of you who wish to clean out your colon but can not obtain the services of a colon therapist, or who want to cleanse within the privacy of your own home, or who simply wish to spend your health-care dollars on organic foods, raw milk, your own education, your emotional work, or simply relaxation, the enema clears out the colon as fully as colon hydrotherapy.

First of all, enemas are not painful. Most people think of enemas as harsh or addictive or medical, and therefore impure or painful. I will say it again: properly done enemas don't cause pain; enemas are safe; enemas, used properly, will assist the colon to work more fully and will not cause the colon to become dependent; enemas are gentle; enemas are safe. In my eight years of working with enemas, I have come to see enemas as a gentle but powerful healing tool.

Enemas Throughout the Ages

Many diverse cultures have used enemas throughout the ages. There are references to the enema in the Bible, as there are in the ancient Egyptian papyruses. An ancient remedy from India, or Ayurvedic culture, incorporates the enema for relief of migraines.

FYI: The article entitled, "Value of Colon Hydrotherapy Verified by Medical Professionals". contains a detailed medical opinions about hydrotherapy. See: www.tldp.com.

Enemas were known in Babylonia, China, and Americas where native Indians used them. In the 17th century, enemas were considered essential to well-being throughout the Western world. In France, enemas were regarded as essential for health; Louis XIV is said to have had thousands of enemas. In the United States, a Dr. Kellogg reported in the *Journal of American Medicine* that in more than 40,000 cases, as a result of diet, exercises, and enema, (in all but twenty cases), he had used no surgery for the treatment of gastrointestinal disease in his patients.

More recently, enemas have been very popular among famous people in the United States and England due to their reputation as a healthy weight loss and beauty aid. It is well known that Demi Moore, Burt Reynolds, Madonna, Kenny Loggins, and Janet Jackson engage in a regular regime of colon cleansing.

Enemas as Tools in Hospitals

Enemas have been and continue to be one of the most important tools used in medical hospitals for the care of patients. On every patient's chart is a list of characteristics to manage; on the top of this patient management list is the daily bowel movement. The medical community sees to it that people in their care move their bowels daily. If a patient doesn't move their bowels daily, treatment is administered to empty the bowels. Unfortunately, due to the influence of pharmaceutical companies and the economical pressures in hospitals today, laxatives are now used most often for emptying the bowels. Before these modern pressures, enemas were the tool of choice. It was hospital nurses who stumbled upon the benefits of using coffee in enemas. And enemas are still used in hospitals today when laxatives and suppositories fail.

Dispelling the Myths About Enemas

I personally have now given thousands of enemas to people who have found that the process of going through a colon cleansing plan reliably brings them relief from headaches, nausea, backaches, bloating and gas, fatigue, IBS, fibromyalgia, chronic sinus infections, and other chronic health imbalances. Enemas do assist people to full health.

Because I have had the great fortune of experiencing firsthand the health benefits of enemas, it is very important to me that the frequent rumors that have been spread about enemas come to an end. A few of these rumors are:

1. **Enemas are not as effective as chemical laxatives, colon hydrotherapy or colon boards.** This is not accurate. Enemas are as effective, and often a healthier choice, than any of the above. Colonics are given priority largely because people haven't learned how to give enemas that are of the same therapeutic value as colon hydrotherapy. Whether or not an enema clears out the entire colon is a matter of skill. Enemas, when administered by a knowledgeable person, are as effective in clearing out the entire length of the colon as any other colon cleansing method. This is why I refer to enemas as therapeutic enemas throughout this book. This is a skill that can easily be learned by you. Additionally, enemas are far more effective and healthier for the body than chemical laxatives. Over time, chemical laxatives will weaken the muscles of the digestive tract, as well as interfere with neural communication.

2. **Enemas are impure and any good feelings from an enema could only involve sexual perversion.** Enemas are wholesome. Enemas are healthy. And enemas do induce a feeling of both physical and psychological refreshment, lightness, relaxation, and even pleasure.

   Gerda Boyesen, a world-renowned clinical psychologist, has come to believe that the colon has other roles than as a passageway for waste materials. She believes that the colon has a dual biological and psychological role. She sees the colon engaged in the vital job of the regulation of physical, emotional, mental, and spiritual health. This function is now known as psycho-peristalsis. Psycho-peristaltic activity can be measured through a stethoscope placed on the abdomen. Restoration via psycho-peristalsis of the instinctive flow of life energy brings homeostasis and self-regulation. This healing function—the

FYI: To learn more of the sad truth of the way in which drug companies are influencing the medical profession, read through www.mercola.com/2000/jul/30/doctors_death.htm and www.citizen.org. In addition, look for Michael Moore's movie about drug companies and their consuming drive for profit. www.michaelmoore.com.

FYI: To read about "psycho-peristalsis," go to Gerda Boyesen's Web site at www.biodynamic. org/clinic.

digestion of the by-products of nervous and emotional stress—is the core of healing in the human body and mind and psyche.

Another example of the mental/emotional influence of the colon comes from the work of endocrinologists. In the last fifteen years, scientists who study our glands and hormones have discovered that serotonin and some forty other neurotransmitters, normally thought of as mood or brain chemicals, all reside overwhelmingly in the intestines rather than the brain (perhaps 95% versus 2%). What these neurotransmitters of the gut point to is a second brain in our gut. Yes, a second brain that is, in part, our colon. This second brain is now referred to as the *enteric nervous system.*

Taking enemas may well be a powerful and effective therapeutic tool for some people. Colon cleansing does seem to positively affect how many people feel about themselves, and about the amount of stress they experience in trying to keep

---

The Truth About Municipal Water

One of the easiest ways to introduce unhealthy microbes into your system is to put impure water directly into your colon. When impurities and parasites go in your mouth, your saliva, your stomach acids, and all your body's defenses have an opportunity to neutralize this toxin or parasite. This is not the case with putting water into the colon. If you use impure water or dirty equipment to give yourself an enema, you are putting your health at risk. "Most Municipal water supplies in the United States are home to protozoa like Giardia and Cryptosporidium; and one in five Americans drinks water that violates federal health standards. Every year, almost a million North Americans become sick from waterborne diseases; and about one percent die."

-Galland, Leo M.D. *Power Healing*, New York, Random House, 1997

---

up with a stressful world, as enemas do seem to stimulate the release of neurotransmitters.

In addition, for many men the prostate is stimulated by the pressure of the solution and the nozzle when an enema is taken. This internal pressure near to the prostate causes pleasure for many men and this is just fine.

In India, an Ayurvedic migraine recipe speaks to the way in which enemas can positively effect areas of the body that are seemingly not even connected to the colon. With the guidance of this recipe, one takes a cleansing enema and then an implant enema with warm sesame oil. It is thought that this treatment ends a headache due to its ability to get the vital essences flowing from the intestinal chakra, where they were stuck, up to the head chakra, where they are needed.

3. **Enemas are addictive and destroy one's own ability to move stool out of the body daily.** I have had the great fortune of working with thousands of clients who have used enemas on a daily, weekly, and monthly basis, over the last six years. Not one of the thousands of people that I have worked with lost any ability that they didn't have before. Using water and other solutions to more fully clear out the colon to reach higher levels of health does not cause the body to function less well.

We must remember that people reach for this tool of colon cleansing because they are constipated, are struggling with a chronic illness such as Irritable Bowel Syndrome or Fibromyalgia or don't desire to be a mortality statistic. (Cardiovascular diseases claimed 931,108 lives in 2001 or, in other words, 38.5 percent of all deaths in 2001 were caused by cardiovascular diseases. Some sources believe that the incidence of this disease will increase by 50% within the next decade.) True, many of these issues have nothing to do with daily bowels movements; but yet again, they do. Cleansing the colon on a schedule that best fits the needs of your individual body always brings improved health.

Buying At-Home Enema Equipment

Although this section contains shameless self-promotion, I decided to add it because I can pass along information about product features that I have learned through trial and error. For readers who have never purchased enema equipment, the following guide offers a description of features that will help you make a decision about what type of enema bag to buy:

Price

Price is an important consideration if you're on a tight budget. The enema bags that I sell online range from $8.50 to $225. The difference in price reflects features such as bag capacity, choices in clamps, and durability. Look for my notes on these topics in the chart that follows.

Bag Capacity

A three to four quart capacity is ideal. Smaller bags will need to be refilled.

Easy or Hard to Clean

This feature is an important consideration because mold can accumulate inside a bag that's not dried properly. Easy cleaning is also an important consideration if you intend to use implants such as essential oils. Oils need to be cleaned off the interior surface of your bag after each use. If the bag has a wide opening, you'll be able to reach inside to clean and dry the inside surface.

Choice of Clamps

Most bags come with a standard plastic clamp that has a multi-position ratchet mechanism. This may be upgraded to an easy-to-use ramp clamp that is purchased separately. A ramp-clamp upgrade is not possible with some bags.

Choice of Nozzle

If you're new to enema equipment, you may not be familiar with a nozzle. It's a molded plastic tip with rounded edges that has several holes to distribute the flow of water. Nozzles are attached to the end of the hose that's used with the enema bag.

Buying on a Budget

If you're on a budget, here are some tips for using the accessories that come with the Red and Blue Fountain enema bags that are listed on the chart in this chapter:

Use the Douche tip Instead of the Pencil-shaped Enema tip

The Red and Blue Fountain bags come with an enema tip that's too small and too hard to use as a nozzle. Use the douche tip instead.

Use the Pencil-shaped Enema tip as a Connector

If you can afford to purchase a colon tube with your enema bag, the pencil-shaped enema tip can be used as a connector to attach a colon tube to the hose. This will add an extra thirty or fifty inches to the hose, and the colon tube will double as a nozzle.

FYI: Just over half of McDonald's roughly 30,000 worldwide units are outside the U.S. Burger King recently opened its first units in Brazil and will soon open its first Chinese unit. Yum's KFC unit arrived in China in 1987, and has since grown to about 1,200 restaurants there.

- Scott Kilman
  Steven Gray
  Wall Street Journal

Length of Hose

Hose length is a consideration for ease-of-use. A longer hose allows you to set up your equipment so that you can see the flow of water. (You can also add a Flowmeter which allows you to monitor the flow of your solution.) Hose length is a consideration if you plan to take your enema in the tub. When you lie on your back in a tub of warm water, you can relax and massage your abdomen while you gradually release the enema liquid into your colon (Note: When your enema is complete, you get out of the tub and release the enema and stool into the toilet).

Colon Tube

Colon tubes have rounded tips that double as nozzles. Colon tubes also add an extra twenty-six inches to the standard length of hose that comes with most enema bags and can deliver the enema solution deeper into the colon.

Enema Bag and Can Material

Enema bags and cans are made out of latex rubber, Indian Rubber, plastic materials, silicone, and stainless steel. Latex,

Bag	Clamp	Nozzle	Cleaning
Traditional Red	Comes with a ratchet hose clamp	Comes with a pencil-shaped enema nozzle and a douche nozzle	Not easy-to-clean
Blue Fountain	Comes with a ratchet hose clamp	Comes with a pencil-shaped enema nozzle and a douche nozzle	Easy-to-clean
Easy Enema	Comes with a ratchet hose clamp	Choice of colon tube or nozzle	Easy-to-clean
2500cc Clear Bag	Custom clamp	Nozzle included	Not easy-to-clean
Flow Master	Comes with a ratchet hose clamp that can be upgraded to a ramp clamp	Optional nozzles: • standard nozzle • colon tube • retention nozzle	Easy-to-clean
Amber, Custom-Made Bag	Comes with a ratchet hose clamp	Nozzle sold separately	Not easy-to-clean
E-Lavage	Comes with a ratchet hose clamp	Retention nozzle and douche nozzle	Not easy-to-clean
Buckets (plastic and stainless steel)	Custom clamp, cannot be modified (plastic)	Hose has a tip that functions as a nozzle (plastic)	Easy-to-clean
Bulb Syringe	Not needed	Comes with a pencil like nozzle	Not easy-to-clean

Capacity	Cost*	Notes
1.5 qts.	$16	The narrow neck and stopper allow this bag to double as a hot water bottle.
1.5 qts.	$16	This smaller-capacity bag has a wide mouth and is an economical choice for people on a budget. This bag will need to be refilled.
2 or 4 qts.	$27 to $39.95	This high-capacity, economical bag has a see-through hose and a choice of nozzles to reduce leakage and deliver solution deeper into the colon. It's long-lasting and can be used with an in-line pump.
2.5 qts.	$14.99	Made of clear plastisol, this bag is used in hospitals and will allow you to see the liquid and monitor your progress.
4 qts.	$144.95 to $225.40	Closest system to colon hydrotherapy. Made of latex or silicone. This bag comes with educational materials.
3 qts.	$75	Attractive custom-made bags made of a stretchable latex with an open top. It is not easy to reach into the bag for cleaning. The transparent color allows you to monitor your water intake. It comes with a chain and an 0-Ring hanging device. Use soap and water only, not recommended with implants.
4 qts.	$50	Comes with traveling case.
1.5 qt. 1.75 qts. and 2.5 qts.	$8.25 to $59	Very economical but slightly clumsy to position because the bucket must stand on a flat surface. Both of these cans are easy-to-use and nontoxic. Stainless steel is the least-toxic material and good for people who are sensitive to plastic. (hose, clamp, and nozzle must be purchased in addition to stainless steel can.)
3-26 ounces	$6 to 37.50	Bulb syringes are made out of PVC plastic and rubber. The small ones are easy to use. The large one is not. Bulb syringes are used for clearing out or implanting into the lower colon.

* Prices subject to change

FYI: For information on the ill effects of distilled water, go to www.mercola.com/article/Diet/water/distilled_water.htm

rubber, and plastic are toxic materials. Many people don't have a direct sensitivity to these materials, but the materials do out gas over time, which causes these materials to end up in the body. If you are chemically sensitive or maintain a zero tolerance for toxins, use stainless steel cans or silicone bags. Even though plastic is a toxic material, it doesn't out gas like rubber. I find it to be inexpensive and nontoxic.

In-Line Pumps

In-line pumps add a therapeutic edge to any enema system. These innovative enema tools will deliver the solution deep into the colon, as they gently push the enema liquid past any blockages. People who use this type of hose and pump system report less cramping, less leaking, and a therapuetic cleansing similar to a professional colon therapy session. The Higginson Syringe, the Smooth Flow Syringe and Hose System are in-line pumps.

How Do I Take Therapeutic Enemas?

First of all, it is important that you not add to your health problems or tax your liver by putting contaminated or chlorinated water into your colon. Chlorine kills good microbes and damages the lining of the colon. I recommend a carbon-based shower filter or, better yet, an under-the-sink reverse osmosis system for a water supply.

Water is so important in the therapeutic enema because it is your main tool for cleaning your colon. A good enema program is when you are able to infuse filtered water deep into your colon to stimulate peristalsis throughout the entire colon, thus cleansing the entire colon and not just the rectal or sigmoid areas. Once enough water is in the colon, you then expel it, and the resulting waste, into the toilet. You then repeat the process one or two more times. This process of taking two to three enemas in a row is called a *therapeutic enema* series. Therapeutic enemas are similar to a simple enema, except for the volume of water you inject and how many times you inject this water in a row.

Don't use a chemical-based enema. Used repeatedly, or in some cases just once, these chemicals irritate the sensitive colonic tis-

The Key to a Successful Enema

You do not need to force yourself to withstand any pain. If you are only able to take a pint of solution before you experience consistent cramping, sit on the toilet and let your bowels empty. You will take more water into your bowels during the next enema. Don't worry if you can only get a little water into your colon. If you have pain for more than twenty to thirty seconds, sit on the toilet. In addition, using any of our Flowmaster systems, the Higginson's Syringe, or the Smooth Flow Syringe with Hose, will allow you to use your equipment to gently move the water out of your sigmoid and rectum deeper into the colon. The key point you need to know in order to take an enema that is the same therapeutic cleanse as a colon hydrotherapy session is that you must get the water beyond the first part of the colon. Most people can take two to four quarts of water into their colon. (Special note: Many people use colon tubes for these same reasons. Colon tubes do work, for some. But there is a larger risk of perforating the colon when you use a colon tube. When you use a syringe pump, you are not at this degree of risk, and you are able to take the solution deeper into your colon.)

FYI: In his book, *The Untold Story of Milk*, author Ron Schmid, N.D., describes an infamous outbreak of salmonella infections in 1985 in the central U.S. that affected approximately 175,000 people, with over 16,000 culture-confirmed cases in what was considered a "multistate" epidemic —all traced to pasteurized milk.

sues. In addition, small amounts of the chemicals end up in your blood stream, which makes more work for your liver. If you are preparing for any kind of colon exam, expertly done enemas are much better for your overall health and will fully clear the colon for the doctors to do their examination or surgery. Mostly, derive a cleansing benefit from filtered water and essential oils, such as peppermint.

Step-by-Step Procedures

Enema bags and buckets are perfect tools for putting water into your colon. These enema containers usually hold between one to six quarts of water. What follows are some simple guidelines for taking a successful therapeutic enema series:

1. Find a Location

Find a comfortable, warm area where you can lie down but where it's also easy for you to get up and get to the toilet. The bathroom floor can be ideal due to the proximity of the toilet. Over the years, I have found that taking an enema series while taking a hot bath works wonders. You are relaxed. Your colon is more able to take larger quantities of water. You can easily clean off after each enema in the series, and your body is in a state of cleansing because of the hot water. Try different locations until you find what works for you. In addition, you will need to know where you will be hanging your bag. You will need a secure place, and the bag will need to be close enough to your body so that the nozzle can gently slide inside your body and also so that you can easily reach the hose clamp. I know many people who find that taking an enema while on their bed, using an IV stand and a rubber sheet, works best for them.

2. Get Acquainted With Your Enema Bag

If this is the first time you have used your bag, play with it a bit before you take your enema. Make sure that you know how the nozzle works, especially if it is a retention nozzle. I recommend retention nozzles for taking larger quantities of water and also for those who leak. Also, if you are using one of the Flowmaster systems, which are expertly designed to deliver enema solutions deeper into the colon, make sure that you understand how the pump system works before you are lying down. Finally, play with the clamp a bit so that you can easily open and close it as you are taking in the desired amounts of solution. This process also allows you a chance to rinse your bag out before using it.

3. Prepare your first enema solution

Before you fill the bag, make sure that the tubing clamp is shut tight so that no water spills out as you are filling the bag. Using plain water often works well. The essential oils, peppermint, rosemary, basil, and frankincense (one to three drops of each) stimulate peristalsis and the immune function. You can try them together or individually. I prefer and recommend them over soap, but if you want to use soap, use one teaspoon to one tablespoon of Dr. Bonner's Hemp Aloe Vera Baby-Mild Pure Castile soap, Peppermint or Lavender soap. When using soaps, use only natural soaps that do not contain any fragrances or petrochemicals. All of the above-mentioned substances will promote a positive musculature response without chemical exposure, and will move your bowels well. Water temperature of 98-104 degrees Fahrenheit is ideal.

4. Find a Place to Hang Your Bag

Hang the bag at least two feet above your body. Three to four feet is even better. Some folks say that hanging the bag too high causes more cramping. This is true only if you let all the water from the bag go into your body during the period of one fill, which I don't recommend and will address in detail soon.

FYI: Mark McAfee's mobile milking barn allows cows to maximize on grazing time and avoid a long walk to a milking barn. At milking time, the mobile unit is moved to a docking site near the grazing cows, and is equipped with its own chiller, milk pump, and generator.

The "I Love You" Massage

One easy way to remember to use massage as a part of an enema is to massage the letters of the phrase " I Love you" on your colon. Starting at beginning of your colon, massage the letter I from the bottom of the ascending colon to the top. After doing this a few times, massage the L from the bottom of the ascending colon and across the transverse colon a few times. Start all over once again with the letter U, massaging from the ascending, across the transverse, and down along the sigmoid colon. You might also try to massage the colon even when not taking your enema. A daily massage helps bowel function. Use castor oil. Along with massage, it can assist the most stubborn colon to put out stool daily.

"Gut function is central to all aspects of health. Correction of abnormalities of gut function must precede and/or accompany the process of healing from any disease. Healthy micro flora and digestive-absorptive function are the basis of restoring and maintaining health."
-John S. Foster, M.D.

---

5. Use a non-petroleum lubricant

Petroleum products always take a toll on your liver. I like Super Salve the best, or a similar plant-based lubricant such as coconut oil. The sterile, water-soluble lubricating jellies such as KY Jelly or Surgilube work well. In this same way, Aloe Vera Gel lubricates well with a therapeutic edge over the latter jellies. Olive oil and vitamin E oil also work, but they don't stay on the nozzle easily.

6. Insert the lubricated nozzle

For insertion, lie on your right side or on your back, which-ever makes insertion easier for you. Make sure that you are comfortable and prepared to spend at least ten minutes taking in the water. (Special Note: For some, time is short. If this is the case, you can still take the enema series. You may find that your colon empties easily and that you don't need to spend the extra time. In other words, don't let a lack of time get in the way of a therapeutic experience.)

7. Open and Close the Clamp

Open the clamp. Five to twenty seconds later, completely close the clamp. This is the most important technique in a deep-cleansing enema. The opening and closing of the clamp keeps you in control of whether or not you will be able to fully clean out your entire colon. Keep the clamp in your hand so that you can, without difficulty, control the flow of water into your body by frequently opening and closing the clamp.

Go slowly! The skill needed for a successful colon cleansing is to let only a small amount of water enter your colon at a time. By a small amount of water, I mean one-half to one cup of water per fill. If you add water too quickly, you will stimulate peristaltic action in the sigmoid and in the rectum, making it nearly impossible to get water all the way into the transverse and ascending colon. If a hint of cramping occurs, immediately stop the flow and relax.

Take a big breath and slowly let it out. Before your session, dap a drop of Peppermint essential oil on your hand or chest. Use the oils to relax by taking deep breaths. I would always have a bottle of Peppermint, Thieves, and Frankincense around while taking enemas to relax and to increase the therapeutic value of the experience. When there is no more cramping, or when thirty to sixty seconds have passed, resume filling your colon with small amounts of solution until your have taken in two to four quarts, or until you can no longer tolerate the amount of cramping that is occurring.

8. Massage Your Abdomen

It can be helpful to gently massage your abdomen to assist the flow of the enema solution into the entire colon. Massage your colon from the bottom-left corner of your abdomen toward your chest, moving the water up the descending colon, then across toward the right, moving the water through the trans-verse colon and finally down the right side into the ascending colon and the cecum area. Reverse the direction of massage when eliminating the enema solution. At the Optimal Health Center, we use a massage tool called a Percussion Massager made by HomeMedic. It works wonders. If you have difficulty holding water or eliminating during a colon cleansing treat-ment, you might try one of these massagers.

9. Filling the Entire Colon

Some people find that being on their left or their right side at some point during a session can make a big difference. Give it a try. Turn over onto your left side and, while gently massag-ing the abdomen, take in more water. This will facilitate fill-ing the entire colon. If you can't take all two to four quarts of water, that's okay. Take only what you can hold comfortably. On the first enema, you are most likely very full of stool in the sigmoid and rectal areas. This is where the nerve endings that stimulate peristalsis are located, so it is very common to only be able to take a small amount of liquid on this first fill. Once you are ready to take the nozzle out and sit on the toilet, make sure that you first closed the clamp.

10. Your Second Enama

After you have expelled your first enema and most of the fecal matter on the toilet, you will want to repeat the procedure.

FYI: Mark McAfee is well-known for his "patho-gen challenge test." A lab in Fresno, California, added 10 million counts of pathogenic bacteria to one liter of his raw milk. The pathogenic bacteria didn't survive. Mark claims that when there is an outbreak of some food-borne illness in the United States, they often blame it on raw milk instead of looking at the real cause of the outbreak.

FYI: In May, 2002, the American Environmental Safety Institute sued chocolate manufacturers in Los Angeles County Court, saying that research showed that dangerous levels of lead and cadmium in chocolate pose a serious health risk, especially to children.

This time follow the same procedure, but now try to increase the volume of water. With your colon less full, you will have room for more water. Taking into your colon one to four quarts of water is key to an effective enema series. And take only as much as you can comfortably hold. Do not put yourself in pain that lasts for more than a few seconds. Use pain as a guide to what your colon is comfortable with. Again, go slowly. On this second enema, you might use Celtic sea salt and Peppermint essential oil, or another essential oil such as Basil or Frankincense or Wheatgrass.

11. Your Third Enema

For your third enema, I recommend that you use one to two quarts of plain filtered water to one cup of brewed enema coffee. Take the coffee enema like you did the first two, but this time hold the solution for a full twelve to fifteen minutes in order to allow the coffee to do its work of stimulating the liver. For more information on the health-giving benefits of coffee enemas, see Implant Recipes in the next chapter.

FYI: Kefir grains die in soy milk and ultra-pasteurized milk.

CHAPTER NINE

Implant Recipes

I rejoice in life for its own sake. Life is no brief candle to me. It is a sort of splendid torch which I have got hold of for the moment; and I want to make it burn as brightly as possible before handing it on to future generations.

- George Bernard Shaw

Implants are therapeutic substances used during or after a colon cleansing session. Implants can be extremely nourishing to the tissues of the colon. Medical doctors have been using anal implants for hundreds of years to get medicine and other healing agents into the body, especially when the person they are administering to is vomiting and can't keep anything down. In other words, enema implants were the original IV fluid.

Using a vinyl bag such as our 2500 cc bag, a 1.5 to 2.0 liter stainless steel can, a Fountain Style enema bag, or a bulb syringe, self-administer your ingredients and leave the solution in your colon for five to thirty minutes. Some solutions are best left in the bowels for hours. These are often not uncomfortable to hold, so you can even go about your daily activities as you retain your implant, or you can lie down and take a nap. Many people find that an implant plug is extremely useful while holding an implant.

The following list is not exhaustive, but rather consists of my favorites. Please do let me know if you are aware of additional implants that you find to be healing. And implants or substances used to stimulate cleansing can also be harmful to the colon. The guideline to follow is to only use the highest-quality and cleanest materials. For instance, always use organic. When implanting butyrate, always use organic, raw grass-fed aged milk.

Coffee Enemas

A coffee enema is used during your third enema in a therapeutic enema series. Coffee enemas became well known through the work of Dr. Max Gerson, M.D., Dr. William Donald Kelley, M.D., and the many heroic people who have struggled with cancer. It is said that coffee enemas were discovered by nurses during war-times who had run out of drugs to relieve soldiers of their pain; there happened to be coffee available that was helping doctors get through the stress. A creative nurse took a risk and added cof-fee to a few enema solutions; the reduction in pain felt by the wounded was dramatic. Coffee enemas are an effective tool for general health and detoxification procedures, and have been found to do an exceptional job of stimulating the liver and gallbladder to release toxins and enhance the liver's filtration process.

Dr. Max Gerson recommended taking a daily coffee enema for two years because the liver is the main organ for the regenera-tion of the body's metabolism for the transformation of food from intake to output.

1. How Does the Coffee Enema Work?

Bile is one of our main bodily fluids used to remove toxins. It is stored in the gallbladder, it draws out environmental and metabolic toxins as well as Candida albicans and other para-site-like organisms. Coffee stimulates the liver to make more bile. (Remember that one needs to eat foods high in cholesterol in order to produce sufficient amounts of bile.) Coffee also stimulates the muscles of the bile ducts in the gallbladder to relax, causing the ducts to open wide, allowing therapeutic amounts of bile, and thus toxins, to pass from the gallbladder into the small intestines.

The neutraceuticals, Theophylline and Theobromine, dilate blood vessels, increasing blood dialysis across the colon wall. This increased blood supply to the intestinal tract improves muscle tone and digestion, as well as the elimination processes. Additionally, given that all of our blood passes through the liver every three minutes, the twelve to fifteen minute coffee retention enema increases blood flow through the liver, resulting in a form of dialysis and a uniquely effective detoxification.

2. Quenching of Free Radicals

The coffee enema increases the production of the enzyme glutathione S-transferase, or GST, by 700 times, resulting in a powerful and effective quenching of free radicals. This blood cleansing process happens because of the action of the palmitic acid in the coffee. Made-for-enemas coffee ought to have a higher level of these Palmitates in the coffee.

As of the year 2004, one in three people had cancer. I have worked with countless cancer clients who swear by the coffee enema. First of all, coffee enemas consistently alleviate pain. In addition, coffee enemas seem to be helpful due to their ability to stimulate the bile ducts to relax and open wide, allowing tumor toxins to pass easily into the small intestines. As tumors break down, proteins are produced and abnormal molecules of the tumor waste are released into the blood, which when not quickly removed can be quite detrimental. By cleaning out the colon and then taking a coffee enema, the body is relieved from these toxic products, thus removing a burden from the metabolic processes of detoxification.

3. Daily Coffee Enemas

For some, daily coffee enemas can make all the difference in the world with levels of pain and with the speed by which one heals. In this program, Ten Days to Optimal Health, I do encourage you to take a coffee enema with every therapeutic enema series. In addition to this level of cleansing, I encourage you to experiment for a few days: take a coffee enema series for a few days in a row. If you feel great afterwards, keep taking one a day. But know that once the body is pretty well detoxified, once the bulk of the healing, the regenerating, and the rebuilding of your body is accomplished, the need for the coffee enemas is no longer present. At that point, the coffee enema can still be used from time to time, as the need arises.

4. Organic, Made-for-Enemas Coffee

Always use organic, made-for-enemas, coffee. Brew four tablespoons of coffee with one quart of water, or one table-

FYI: Sally Fallon has taught us that the Aztecs knew that nuts and seeds have enzyme inhibitors that interfere with digestion. They soaked nuts and seeds in salt water and then put them out in the sun to dry. If nuts and seeds are soaked overnight in salt water, this takes care of the enzyme inhibitors. After nuts and seeds have been soaked overnight (for six to eight hours), they can be placed in a baking dish and dried at a low heat in an oven to make them crispy.

spoon per cup. When the mixture is cool, pour one tablespoons to one cup of the coffee into your enema bag along with one quart of filtered water. Save the extra coffee in a glass jar for your next enema series. Take the solution into your body and retain it for a minimum of twelve full minutes and a maximum of fifteen minutes. Given that you just fully cleaned out the colon with the previous therapeutic enemas, this task ought to be easy. Sit on the toilet and expel. Since the coffee solution is actually absorbed into the hemorrhoidal vein in the sigmoid colon area, and then taken up to the liver by the portal vein, and since the coffee enema needs to be held for twelve to fifteen minutes, many find that using a colon tube as your nozzle not only delivers the coffee solution deeper into the colon, but also makes holding the coffee enemas easier.

5. Using a Colon Tube

In order to use a colon tube, please take care to use the following guidelines:

- Most people find that colon tubes are invaluable. When taking a coffee enema for colon cleansing, it can help to use a 30 colon tube, FR 28, 32 or 34. My highest recommendation is a 30, 32 FR silicone colon tube; silicone is nontoxic, unlike the rubber colon tubes.

- Colon tubes help to deliver the coffee enema higher into the colon where it is able to exert its action most effectively on the liver. Never force a colon tube. Given that you are going to be guiding a colon tube deep into your colon, it is important that you use a food-based lubricant. Super salve is the lubricant of choice. There are many natural herbal ointments available from health food stores. Also, natural oils such butter can be used. Again, never force a colon tube.

6. Extra Tips

How the colon tube is inserted varies between individuals. Here are some helpful tips:

- By no means force a colon tube.

The Butyrate Detoxx Enema

Clearing bowels and stimulating the flushing of the gall-bladder is vital to the successful implementation of detoxification processes. Butyrate, electrolyte, and organic coffee form a potent cleansing solution for the bowels and stimulate contraction of the gall bladder.

Recipe
Combine for enema:
One cup fresh-made organic coffee
Contents of five capsules of butyrate E-Lyte"

The medical doctors in this book recommend that you take this implant enema as often as once a week.

There is evidence to suggest that the metabolism of butyrate—the major fatty acid fuel source for the epithelial cells lining the colon—is impaired in ulcerative colitis. Studies on humans suggest that topical treatment using sodium butyrate may reverse symptoms in ulcerative colitis. Several reports on the use of butyrate enemas for the treatment of distal ulcerative colitis have appeared in the literature. One study showed a striking increase in colon cell mucin synthesis when butyrate was added to standard nutrient medium. The therapeutic effect of butyrate on colitis may be due to its ability to boost the rate of mucin synthesis and restore the colon's mucous lining. Butyrate enemas are prescribed by alternative medicine doctors for the treatment of Crohn's disease and colitis.

FYI: It's important to understand that cleansing is a critical body function. Although the body has built-in mechanisms that cleanse our tissues, enemas are an extremely effective way to augment what the body does naturally.

- Before you insert the colon tube, lay it out on a flat surface. Take note of its natural curve. As you insert the colon tube, slide it into your colon so that this natural curve corresponds with the curve of your colon.

- The best way to insert a colon tube is to begin a flow of water after you have inserted the colon tube a few inches and then to create a channel by further inserting the colon tube in stages, gradually.

FYI: Instructions for forming a Weston A. Price
Foundation chapter in
your city maybe found
on the local chapters
page on the Weston A.
Price Foundation Web
site: westonaprice.org/
localchapters

The Butyrate Detoxx Enema (continued)

Understand that healing is an art. I, too, am learning daily
about the tools of this art. The above-mentioned is one of
those tools that I am offering you as a fellow artist, rather
than as an expert. In this vein, drinking raw, grass-fed,
milk is excellent for these very reasons. And in this vein,
it is possible that using aged, raw, grass-fed milk inside
the colon could improve your health tremendously.

- I recommend a medium-diameter colon tube, French 28 to
  32, although I do have many clients who swear by the thinner colon tubes.

- Each person reacts differently to colon tubes, even when a
  channel of enema water or solution is created. You might
  never get the tube all the way in, and you should NEVER
  force the tube.

- It is not really necessary to get the colon tube all the way
  in to accomplish a high enema. Use time, patience, and
  gravity to your benefit. Unless your colon is congenitally
  abnormal, the enema should be able to reach the high areas
  of the colon by taking at least two quarts of water.

- Most likely, the best way to take a deep colon tube insertion is to start out on your left side, take some tube and
  water, and then after the tube is in about 10+ inches, turn
  over on your back, with hips elevated on a pillow or something. It's better to have someone else helping, but that's
  not possible for most people. Just remember that it's not
  necessarily how deep the colon tube goes in but, rather,
  how deep the water goes in that really counts. This takes
  time, relaxation and listening to one's own body.

Olive Oil/Aloe Vera Implant/MSM

An excellent recipe for healing the colon is a mixture of olive oil,
aloe vera, and MSM. In an enema bag or syringe, pour one-half
to one cup of organic olive oil and one-half to one cup of organic

aloe vera juice. (Special Note: Oil will deteriorate latex over time.) Open four MSM capsules and empty into mixture (approx. 4000 mg total). Mix as well as you can. Once you have the implant inside your colon, massage your colon from left to right. To move the implant further into your colon, use a colon tube or gently lift up into a shoulder stand, if this is comfortable for you, to help your body move the implant farther along into your colon. Try to retain the implant for at least thirty minutes. You may find that you can comfortably retain it for many hours. This recipe works well because it heals the colon tissue while it assists the colon in functioning more fully. I must warn you though: it can be messy.

FYI: Membership in the Weston A. Price Foundation includes quarterly issues of *Wise Traditions* Magazine.

Bifidobacterium bifidum

More and more health professionals are realizing that implanting dairy-free bifidum bacteria into the colon facilitates optimal health. Bifidum stimulates an environment that discourages harmful bacteria and yeasts by taking away their home along the intestinal walls. Bifidum bacteria produce lactic and acetic acids that help to maintain a healthy intestinal tract. Bifidum bacteria produce B vitamins to assist the large intestine in processing food naturally and efficiently. Start out with one to two teaspoons of this probiotic in eight to ten ounces of water, organic aloe juice or raw, grass-fed, whey. You may increase the dosage up to two tablespoons over time. Bifidum is placed in the colon after the colon hydrotherapy session or the enema series and is held as long as you are able to hold it. It is important to note here that it is not acidophilus that is implanted into the colon, as that species of bacteria largely resides in the small intestine. (Although I do recommend that some people take a probiotic daily, especially those folks who aren't eating large amounts of fermented foods daily.)

Human Fecal Matter

At the Probiotic Therapy Research Center, doctors are using human probiotic infusions to establish normal health flora. I have had a few clients work with these tools, but as of this edition of *Ten Days*, I do not have an opinion of its effectiveness. See www. probiotictherapy.com.au/ for more information.

FYI: Changes in agriculture are raising new questions regarding the rights of all rural Americans. Historically, farmers have defended their "right to farm," whenever residential development has brought in urban neighbors with no appreciation for the normal sights, sounds, and smells of farming.

More recently, rural residents have claimed their "right of self-defense" against growing threats to their health, safety, and welfare brought on by new industrial farming methods, particularly large-scale confinement animal-feeding operations (CAFOs).

- John Ikerd
 Small Farm Today Magazine

Butyrate

The colonic mucosa is highly dependent upon the presence of luminal nutrients. This dependence is most marked in the sigmoid and rectal sections of the colon. The major luminal nutrients are short-chain fatty acids that are produced as a by-product of colonic fermentation of carbohydrates. Butyrate appears to be the short-chain fatty acid most avidly metabolized by the colonic mucosa. The only natural source of butyrate is in raw, grass-fed cow's milkfat. Up to 10% of milk's fatty acids appear to be butyric acid. It is in this form that butyrate can be transmitted directly to the body. Preliminary studies suggest that butyrate may be effective in the treatment of colon cancer. To show the growing interest in using butyrate in the colon, I will take a recipe from the book, *The Detoxx Book, Detoxification of Biotoxins in Chronic Neurotoxin Syndrome* by John S Foster, M.D., et. al.:

Wheat Grass Enema

Ann Wigmore popularized the use of wheatgrass juice implants. Today, many people have used these implants to recover their health. Using an implant syringe to implant one to two ounces. of fresh wheatgrass juice and one to two cups of water into the colon nourishes the body with chlorophyll, vitamins, and minerals in a more effective way than any multivitamin will.

Epsom salts

Before surgery became the tool of choice in hospitals, Epsom salts and coffee enemas were used to deal with gallbladder problems. These methods were hugely successful. Add 1 tablespoon of Epsom salts per quart of filter water to your enema bag, along with two to four tablespoons of brewed, organic, made-for-enema, coffee. The Epsom salts cause the head of the gallbladder to relax so that stone can be released into your bile duct to allow gallstones to leave your gallbladder along with bile. Along with an excellent diet, lots of grass-fed butter, and a bit of olive oil, you can fully address your gall bladder needs with this enema implant.

In addition, Epsom salts in the enema water work to relax the colon. For those of you who struggle to hold any amount of water, using Epsom salts in water as your solution can work wonders.

Glycerin

Glycerine is a commonly used suppository for relief of constipation. When you find that you aren't able to evacuate with a plain water, peppermint-water, or soap water enema, use one to two tablespoons of glycerine in your enema water.

Flax-seed tea

Flax-seed tea, instead of water, provides an enema that is soothing rather than irritating. The essential fatty acids of the tea work to protect the cellular membranes of the colon. I recommend the use of flax-seed tea enemas if you take regular enemas.

Recipe

1-3 quarts of filtered water.

Do not boil. Heat the water only to the point where it is still comfortable to touch the water without scalding your finger. You do not want to destroy the heat-sensitive fats within the seeds. Add one tablespoons of organic flax seeds to the water. Soak for 30 minutes. Keep your eye on the solution. If it begins to thicken, drain the water off the seeds before 30 minutes is up. Take this solution as your second or third enema in the series. You could add your coffee to this enema, if you wish.

Green Tea

Phenols, an antioxidant that has antitumor effects, has been show to slow cancer cell growth. If you have a family history of colon cancer or prostate cancer, using green tea in your enema regime is an excellent idea. I recommend that you take an enema series to fully clean out the colon. Once the colon is empty, take in two to six cups of brewed, organic green tea into your colon as an implant. Hold the solution for as long as you are able. If at any point you have cramping, empty your colon.

Slippery Elm

Steep one tablespoon of Slippery Elm bark with two cups of water. Strain out the bark. Implant into colon. This mixture will neutralize an acid colon and absorb foul gases. It is very soothing and can be helpful with colitis, diarrhea, and hemorrhoids.

FYI: The U.S. Department of Agriculture estimates that this year farmers will pay $8.2 billion for petroleum, up 21% from two years ago. Adding in the cost of fertilizers and pesticides (which are derived from petroleum and natural gas products), and electricity, farmers are expected to pay more for energy-related items for the third consecutive year.

- USA Today

FYI: Wander down the aisles of most American grocery stores and you'll find a surprising choice of foods from foreign countries—ripe blackberries from Mexico, capers from Morocco, hearts of palm from Costa Rica, and sweet peppers from South Africa. The list goes on.

While all these foreign imports may be a boon for consumers, they're one reason the once-huge U.S. agricultural trade surplus is rapidly deflating. It's down from $ 9.6 billion just last year to only a projected $1 billion in 2005, raising the possibility of a deficit in the future.

How could the world's breadbasket be staggering when it comes to a traditional strength like the American farm? The question comes at an awkward moment as overall U.S. trade deficits hit record highs of more than $ 600 billion a year.

The answer is a culinary tale involving changing consumer tastes, expanding global farm output, and the subsidies governments offer a politically sensitive industry.

- Katherine Dillin
  *Christian Science
  Monitor*

Sesame Oil and Herbs

In the tradition of Ayurvedic enemas, a sesame oil implant is the preferred method of addressing the issue of therapeutic enemas or basti. It is thought that the stomach should be emptied and that the best time to take the enema is in the morning or the evening. The usual procedure for basti is first to introduce five ounces of warm (not hot) sesame oil into the rectum and retain it for 10 minutes. Then, without expelling the oil, introduce a mixture of oil and herbal tea and retain it for at least 30 minutes. The mixture should consist of another 5 ounces of sesame oil, mixed with 16 ounces (1 pint) of tea made from herbs steeped in hot water, and then strained and cooled to about body temperature.

The herbs to use are an Indian herb called dashamoola (which can be found at most alternative pharmacies or natural food stores) or licorice root. After you hold the solution for the suggested time, sit on the toilet and allow the passage of the liquid and stool. This treatment is excellent for those with a dry colon, as it lubricates, as well as cleanses, the colon. The herbs offer relief from a wide range of illnesses such as ulcerative colitis and arthritis. In my center, I use sesame-oil implants with excellent results for people who are chronically constipated.

Essential Oils

Using essential oils inside of the colon is an exciting and growing practice. Essential oils are volatile liquids that ideally are extracted through distillation. The oils are taken from flowers, seeds, leaves, stems, bark and root of herbs, bushes, and trees. The essential oil of a plant is the plant's healing force and it functions in the plant as the chemical defense system. Because of their antibacterial, antifungal and antiviral properties, essential oils are able not only to provide excellent health and cleansing benefits to humans, but they also enhance immune function and balance out the hormones.

Not all essential oils are of the same quality. Be careful with which brand of essential oils you choose to put inside your body. Always start with a small amount of the oil. I have given a few recipes below that I have used with great results. Please be aware that the oils work differently for different people, so you might find that you need to change the recipe. Also, since this is a growing practice, you will want to keep learning what others are discovering.

Peppermint

This oil is a much healthier alternative to stimulating peristalsis in the colon than is soap. Add to water during your therapeutic enemas. Using two to three drops of peppermint per quart of filtered water in your first and/or second enema in the series can increase the therapeutic effectiveness of your colon cleansing.

Lavender

Implant two to six drops of lavender with one cup of olive oil after a colon cleansing session. Studies have shown that lavender inhibits the incidence of adenocarcinomas of the colon in rats. Lavender has been shown to increase the rate of wound healing. As an implant, lavender works wonders for anal fissures, hemorrhoids, chronic headaches and nausea, difficult menstrual cycles, and more.

Frankincense and Myrrh

Frankincense and Myrrh are supportive of the prostate. Myrrh has hormone-like properties and is anti-inflammatory. Frenincense heals the prostate. There are many natural doctors worldwide who are using essential oils to assist with prostrate issues. The Optimal Health Center has an essential oil, raw goat milk soap that has been developed for the prostate.

Thieves

Thieves is one of the many blends of essential oils that have been put together by the Young Living Essential Oils company. It was created from research about a group of 15th-century thieves who rubbed oils on themselves to avoid contracting the plague while they robbed the bodies of the dead and dying. This blend of therapeutic-grade essential oils was tested at Weber State University for its potent antimicrobial properties. Thieves was found to have a 99.96 percent kill

FYI: The busiest McDonald's restaurant in the world is not in America but thousands of miles away in Pushkin Square. The store serves 30,000 customers a day, as busy as on opening day, January 31, 1990. The menu is essentially the same as in the United States, with the addition of cabbage pie, among other traditional Russian food items.

- New York Times

rate against airborne bacteria. (*Essential Oils Desk Reference*, Essential Science Publishing) Use it on your hands and around your neck before and after giving yourself an enema. If you are a colon hydrotherapist or you are helping out your friend with his or her colon cleansing program, do the same.

Raw Milk and Molasses

There are many poisons in the world we live that are ingested and lodge in the bowel. These must be cleaned to return the body to health and allow natural healing to take place. Milk and molasses enemas cause a lot of bowel action that you will feel as cramps. While cramps are unpleasant, they show the bowel is cleaning itself and that is good. The distress of the cleaning action is overcome by the benefits of moving toxins out of the body. Use three cups of fresh, raw milk and one-half cup of pure molasses. Heat this to body temperature. This solution must be administered quickly as cramps will come quick. The best position for the implant is a head down, knees to chest position. This encourages the implant to flow deep into bowel. For initial treatment, you will want to have a lot of cramping to release build up of toxins. After you release the milk and molasses solution on the toilet, you can follow up with a made-for-enema soap and water enema.

Note: This treatment should only be done with the guidance of a trained health professional as it does cause pain. For instance, I work with a man whose work is disaster relief. He is constantly in contact with chemicals such as asbestos, glass wool, and countless others. He needs his bowel to work hard to remove toxins.

CHAPTER TEN
Supportive Case Studies

Alternative therapies that help us contact the regenerative powers that lie within us, that help us take care of ourselves and prevent disease, and that give us greater control over our lives have a major role to play in the future of health care, and in the healing of our society.

– John Robbins, Reclaiming Our Health

Every new idea, because it is new, must stand up to scrutiny and real-life challenges. The Optimal Health Plan must also hold up under real-life application and for that reason I felt that sharing background information on some of my most definitive clinical case studies is appropriate. Remember, always consult your medical doctor before trying any health plan.

Injury Induced Bowel Problems

One of the most exciting cases involved a young man faced with continual and severe pain throughout his entire body and extreme bowel irregularities:

Case: William, age 42, December 1999

Background: William injured his back at work in 1991. Since that time he has had persistent back pain, and had found that on many days it was hard to walk. His health was being managed poorly through drugs, with subsequent unpleasant side effects. He had a lack of appetite, nausea, and irregular bowel movements, including painful diarrhea. Exercise was not possible due to pain. The back pain had radiated into the groin area so that sex was impossible. Due to his physical health, his psychological health

FYI: As demand for organic food grows, so does the number of organic farmers. Sales of organic food are growing about 18% a year, with meat and fish experiencing the fastest growth, according to figures from the Organic Trade Association. The amount of U.S. certified organic cropland for corn, soybeans, and other major crops doubled from 1997 to 2001, according to the USDA.

- Janet Adamy
  Wall Street Journal

had dropped to the point where he was having daily panic attacks. He was frustrated and angry for not being able to find help.

Sessions and Treatment Recommendations: He sought out the Optimal Health Center despite the fears of his family due to his chronic constipation. At the first session, he spent a great deal of time explaining what he was going through, including what he ate, drank, and took by way of drugs. We did a colon hydrotherapy session that lasted for 15 minutes the first time. William was an extremely picky eater. I got him to cut out all the alcohol, sugar, and grains. He would eat only chicken, fish, eggs, raw milk, olive oil, asparagus, and broccoli, for the most part. He also drank a tremendous amount of water. I was able to supplement his diet with Living Fuel, l-glutamine, magnesium, cod liver oil, a daily lemon, Super Aloe, and MSM. He had a weekly colon therapy session.

Status (March, 2002): William now has normal bowel movements one to two times a day without medication. He is no longer throwing up. His anxiety attacks have gone away. He still experiences pain in his back, but not throughout his whole body. If he stretches and gets regular massage, the pain is almost gone. Groin pain has decreased and seems to be getting better. He is exercising everyday with minimal discomfort.

Fibromyalgia and Emotional Stress

According to the American College of Rheumatology, three to six million Americans have fibromyalgia and ninety percent of the cases of fibromyalgia occur in women. This case demonstrates how toxicity in the body can cause pain and emotional problems.

Case: Joyce, age 40, October 2001

Background: Joyce presented herself at the clinic with fibromyalgia, chronic fatigue, irritable bowel, a spastic bladder, intense carbohydrate cravings, anxiety, depression, a sleep disorder, and severe mood swings. Her bowels were moving only one to three times per week. Her mood and temper were at times extreme.

Sessions and Treatment Recommendations: During each of her weekly sessions, our work together included reviewing her eating habits. Originally, her meals consisted of cereal or toast for breakfast, a sandwich at lunch, meat and vegetables for dinner, and fruit smoothies and bread sticks for snacks. Each time I saw her, we would fine-tune her diet.

In her first colon hydrotherapy session, she removed 20 feet of stored stool in a 40-minute period. The bowel issues were taken care of within 35 days by using the OHC plan. Plus, her long-term nutritional habits were refined and brought into sync with her lifestyle needs. She found that raw, grass-fed butter made a tremendous difference in her cravings for carbohydrates as well as in how she felt emotionally. She ate the equivalent of a stick of butter daily. Supplements were used to help her with the other problems; magnesium, an antioxidant, raw, organic liver, a probiotic, and cod liver oil.

This first round of treatments got her feeling 50% better. Three months later, after two fasts, she finally regulated her sleep schedule and was able to cry and rage a lot. She now spent 90% of her days with no pain. She has had to maintain a strict diet to keep her symptoms from flaring up. Her anxiety and depression were completely gone and she found that if she gave herself permission to cry when she felt like it, she quickly moved through any mood swings.

Status (December, 2002): Approximately 90% of her problems are gone as she continues to maintain her new eating habits, to practice emotional release, and to take her supplements.

Candida and Infertility

If the body is provided with optimal nutrition, it has a remarkable ability to heal itself. This case illustrates the rejuventative power of whole food.

Case: Louisa, age 27, weight 190, May 1999

Background: Louisa presented herself to me with irritable bowel, migraines, infertility issues, no menses, seasonal allergies,

FYI: If your diet is too low in cholesterol, you may lose your ability to make hormones that are critical for good health. For example, hormones help you deal with stress and regulate the levels of glucose in the body.

Endometriosis, swollen glands, brain fog, and teeth-grinding, in addition to which, she was overweight. She also had erratic bowels movements one to five times per day. Her eating habits were very bad and her intake consisted of fruit, coffee, donuts and cereal for breakfast; sandwiches, chips, and beans for lunch; potatoes, fish, and soy products for dinner; and cookies, fruit, soda, and ice cream for snacks.

Session and Treatment Recommendations: Louisa was very excited about changing her diet because she knew it was imbalanced and she very much wanted to have a baby. I started her immediately on the OHC Plan. She drank a lot of raw milk for its high vitamin A content to enhance fertility. She removed very little from her colon in the first session. Subsequent sessions were very successful.

After completion of the 35-day plan, she continued with colon therapy for three more months, having three sessions a month. She also continued following the OHC plan diet to the letter for these three months. We set up an exercise plan at about the two month mark, which for the first time in her life she was able to follow faithfully due to how good she felt about herself. The supplements she took included magnesium, grape seed extract, an antifungal rotation, and fermented kefir. She also eliminated all the mold that was present in her house.

Status (November, 2002): Today, Louisa has lost a total of 43 pounds. She has two healthy bowel movements a day, and no signs of Irritable Bowel Syndrome, migraines, teeth-grinding, swollen glands, or brain fog. Her period returned on a regular monthly schedule after six months. Her seasonal allergies are no longer a problem unless she eats pasteurized dairy, sugar, or wheat products. After 2 ½ years of finding and maintaining her optimal health level she is well … and now has a very healthy six-month old son.

Anal Fissures

An anal fissure is a painful condition in which the lining of the rectum is torn. It is caused by constipation or a forced bowel movement. Once the lining is torn, each subsequent bowel movement is painful, and the pain is often accompanied by bleeding.

Case: Joseph, early 50s, April 2002

Background: The following client sought conventional medical treatment and was examined by doctors, yet nothing was diagnosed. So after more inquiries, a surgeon was recommended as an option. But after two consultations with the surgeons, he got scared off by the prospects and the problems involved. As his pain and bleeding increased, he researched the Web and finally self-diagnosed a classical anal fissure. With this information and a consult with a new doctor, he finally got confirmation of his diagnosis. For two years, he used prescription cortisone creams and other ointments. Cortisone relieved the pain, but cured nothing. All mineral-based ointments did nothing but further agitate the fissure. One day, a friend he discussed this problem with recommended a holistic approach and possibly seeing a colon therapist. This brought him to our center and to a solution to his problem. By the time I was working with him, he had an anal fissure that for six years had slowly grown into a severe problem causing extreme discomfort and anxiety. He was unable to sit down for any length of time and was at his wits end.

Sessions and Treatment Recommendations: This client was hesitant to follow the Ten Day Plan to the letter, so we improvised. I recommended that he use a combination of nutrition, herbal medicine and timely colon hydrotherapy, plus self-administered enemas to heal the fissures. His eating habits were in need of change, as well. For his new diet, he added fruits daily, ate more green vegetables, and ate only rice, spelt, and quinoa for his grains. Joseph also stayed away from chocolate, coffee, alcohol, and pasteurized dairy for the better part of two months. Besides the deeper benefits of colon cleansing, the hydrotherapy gave him a clean rectal area and a break from the strains of defecation. He took an enema every other day and an enema implant every fourth day, for about six months, until the fissure was completely healed. He used the enema implant recipe using aloe vera, olive oi,l and MSM that soothed the area and promoted healing.

FYI: The Kombucha e-Group on Yahoo offers a lively discussion on a variety of kombucha-related topics.

I also had him use Super Salve as a topical treatment that would prevent fissure swelling and infection. The Super Salve was applied to the area two times a day.

Status (February, 2004): Joseph has torn the fissure during defecation only once in the last year. But this healed up quickly with a renewal of his OHC plan for two weeks. Otherwise, except for some occasional itching, he has been free of pain and bleeding, and has been able to pass occasional hard stools. He has also been able to moderately drink alcohol and eat chocolate and he has eliminated the use of any medications. Basically, today he feels good and enjoys life!

Diabetes, Obesity, and Candida

After one week on the OHC plan, most people experience a noticeable shift in their energy level that helps them with their decisions regarding lifestyle changes. This next case is an example.

Case: Martha, 59, weight 259 lbs, September 1999

Background: Martha's excessive weight of 259 lbs. was a big concern of hers, as were her diabetes, high cholesterol level, and an overgrowth of Candida. These problems caused Martha daily pain, three to four watery bowel movements per day and they largely limited her activities to her home. She had tried all types of diet plans without success. Her goals were to get off Glyburide for diabetes, eliminate her pain, lose weight, and detoxify her system.

Treatment Recommendations: Martha went through the 35-day plan with great success. The first week she became quite ill. Once she got through the first week, she started to feel energetic, which inspired her to continue. She lost three to six pounds per week. Instead of being in constant pain, she was only in pain for short periods throughout the week. She continued the OHC plan, switching to a monthly colon hydrotherapy session. She fasted every three to four months. During the fasts, she would do three colon hydrotherapy sessions. She drinks Living Fuel daily. Her supplement program included olive leaf extract, magnesium, calcium, cod liver oil, DHEA, B6, B complex, chlorella, CoQ10, and a probiotic formula. She also gave herself a weekly essential oil implant.

Status (October, 2002): Martha now weighs 169 lbs. and is off all medications. She mainly sticks with the OHC plan (but eats pie or something similar a couple times a month as a treat). Her body pain is largely gone except when she doesn't stretch and the day after she eats pie. Her cholesterol levels are normal. She is very pleased with herself and is experiencing a much fuller life.

FYI: To add fizz to your kombucha, leave a bottle out at room temperature for a few days before drinking it.

FYI: The Maasai in Kenya are nomads who consume mostly milk and meat. They show little evidence of heart disease.

FYI: The French consume saturated fat and cholesterol, yet they have low coronary heart-disease rates.

REFERENCES

1. Effect of butyrate enemas on the colonic mucosa in distal ulcerative colitis. Scheppach W, Sommer H, Kirchner T, Paganelli GM, Bartram P, Christl S, Richter F, Dusel G, Kasper H. *Gastroenterology.* 1992 Jul;103(1):51-6.

    These data support the view that butyrate deficiency may play a role in the pathogenesis of distal ulcerative colitis and that butyrate irrigation ameliorates this condition.

2. Protective role of probiotics and prebiotics in colon cancer. Ingrid Wollowski, Gerhard Rechkemmer and Beatrice L Pool-Zobel. *American Journal of Clinical Nutrition*, Vol. 73, No. 2, 451S-455s, February 2001

    In conclusion, colon cancer, which in a high proportion of the population is due to somatic mutations occurring during the lifetime of an individual, could be retarded or prevented by preventing these mutations. LAB and probiotics that enhance LAB have been shown to deactivate genotoxic carcinogens.

3. Protection from gastrointestinal diseases with the use of probiotics. Philippe R Marteau, Michael de Vrese, Christophe J Cellier and Jürgen Schrezenmeir. *American Journal of Clinical Nutrition*, Vol. 73, No. 2, 430S-436s, February 2001.

    Accumulating research evidence suggests that probiotics may have a role in human therapies.

4. Saturated fats: what dietary intake? J Bruce German and Cora J Dillard. *American Journal of Clinical Nutrition*, Vol. 80, No. 3, 550-559, September 2004.

    Unfortunately, the overwhelming emphasis on the role of saturated fats in the diet and the risk of CAD has distracted investigators from studying any other effects that individual saturated fatty acids may have on the body. If saturated fatty acids were of no value or were harmful to humans, evolution would probably not have established within the mammary gland the means to produce saturated fatty acids—butyric, caproic, caprylic, capric, lauric, myristic, palmitic, and stearic acids—that provide a source of nourishment to ensure the growth, development, and survival of mammalian offspring.

Butyrate is a well-known modulator of genetic regulation, and it also may play a role in cancer prevention. Published information thus far indicates that butyric acid exhibits contradictory and paradoxical behavior. Although butyric acid is an important energy source for the normal colonic epithelium, is an inducer of the growth of colonic mucosa, and is a modulator of the immune response and inflammation, it also functions as an antitumor agent by inhibiting growth and promoting differentiation and apoptosis.

5. Membrane peroxidation by lipopolysaccharide and iron-ascorbate adversely affects Caco-2 cell function: beneficial role of butyric acid. Frederic Courtois, Ernest G Seidman, Edgard Delvin, Claude Asselin, Sandra Bernotti, Marielle Ledoux and Emile Levy. *American Journal of Clinical Nutrition*, Vol. 77, No. 3, 744-750, March 2003.

   Bacterial endotoxin and prooxidants may overwhelm antioxidant defenses and become deleterious to enterocyte function, whereas butyric acid and BHT may provide antioxidant protection.

6. Colostrum and milk-derived peptide growth factors for the treatment of gastrointestinal disorders. Raymond J Playford, Christopher E Macdonald and Wendy S Johnson. *American Journal of Clinical Nutrition*, Vol. 72, No. 1, 5-14, July 2000

   In summary, research examining the potential benefits of using recombinant peptides or colostral-derived preparations for a wide range of gastroenterologic conditions is underway. Early results are encouraging and we envisage the standard use of these products in the clinical management of gastrointestinal diseases within the next decade.

7. Vitamin D status in children, adolescents, and young adults with Crohn disease. Timothy A Sentongo, Edisio J Semaeo, Nicolas Stettler, David A Piccoli, Virginia A Stallings and Babette S Zemel. *American Journal of Clinical Nutrition*, Vol. 76, No. 5, 1077-1081, November 2002

   Division of Gastroenterology, Hepatology, and Nutrition, Children's Memorial Hospital, Northwestern University, Chicago (TAS), and the Division of Gastroenterology and Nutrition, The Children's Hospital of Philadelphia, University of Pennsylvania, Philadelphia (TAS, EJS, NS, DAP, VAS, and BSZ).

   In this sample of pediatric patients with CD, hypovitaminosis D was common and was associated with the winter season, African American ethnicity, CD confined to the upper gastrointestinal tract, and magnitude of lifetime exposure to glucocorticoid therapy. The occurrence of these factors should prompt assessment of 25(OH)D status and clinical care optimized by supplementing subjects who have low serum concentrations.

8. Comparison of monounsaturated fatty acids and carbohydrates for lowering plasma cholesterol. SM Grundy. *New England Journal of Medicine*, Vol. 314:745-748, March 20, 1986, Number 12

Therefore, in short-term studies in which liquid diets are used and body weight is kept constant, a diet rich in monounsaturated fatty acids appears to be at least as effective in lowering plasma cholesterol as a diet low in fat and high in carbohydrates.

FYI: Most people with heart disease have low to moderate levels of cholesterol.

9. Elevated diet-induced thermogenesis and lipid oxidation rate in Crohns disease. Geltrude Mingrone, Esmeralda Capristo, Aldo V Greco, Guiseppe Benedetti, Andrea De Gaetano, Pietro A Tataranni and Giovanni Gasbarrini. *American Journal of Clinical Nutrition,* Vol. 69, No. 2, 325-330, February 1999.

   Patients with inactive ileal CD had significantly higher DIT and lipid oxidation rate than do healthy volunteers. These results may explain why CD patients have difficulty maintaining adequate nutritional status, and the findings also suggest that a diet relatively rich in fat may attain better energy balance.

10. Butyric acid from the diet: actions at the level of gene expression. Smith JG, Yokoyama WH, German JB. *Crit Rev Food Sci Nutr.* 1998 May;38(4):259-97.

    A number of components present in the diet, although nutritionally nonessential, have been discovered to have beneficial effects toward both general health and disease prevention/protection. One such nutrient, butyric acid, can be derived in large quantities from bacterial fementation of dietary fiber in the bowel and is also a component of bovine milk. In particular, butyric acid's ability to modify nuclear architecture and induce death by apoptosis in colon cancer cells is arousing great interest.

11. Probiotics: effects on immunity. Erika Isolauri, Yelda Sütas, Pasi Kankaanpää, Heikki Arvilommi and Seppo Salminen. *American Journal of Clinical Nutrition*, Vol. 73, No. 2, 444S-450s, February 2001

    In conclusion, these data point to the conclusion that probiotics can be used as innovative tools for treating dysfunctions of the gut mucosal barrier, including acute gastroenteritis, food allergy, and inflammatory bowel disease.

12. Effect of a gluten-free diet on gastrointestinal symptoms in celiac disease. Joseph A Murray, Tureka Watson, Beverlee Clearman and Frank Mitros. *American Journal of Clinical Nutrition*, Vol. 79, No. 4, 669-673, April 2004.

    With a gluten-free diet, patients have substantial and rapid improvement of symptoms, including symptoms other than the typical ones of diarrhea, steatorrhea, and weight loss.

13. Saturated fat prevents coronary artery disease? An American paradox. Robert H Knopp and Barbara M Retzlaff. *American Journal of Clinical Nutrition*, Vol. 80, No. 5, 1102-1103, November 200

    In conclusion, the hypothesis-generating report of Mozaffarian et al draws attention to the different effects of diet on lipoprotein physiology and car-

FYI: The cholesterol theory that says saturated fat causes heart disease is easy to disprove:

- animal fat consumption has decreased since 1900.

- Heart disease has increased.

diovascular disease risk. These effects include the paradox that a high-fat, high saturated-fat diet is associated with diminished coronary artery disease progression in women with the metabolic syndrome, a condition that is epidemic in the United States. This paradox presents a challenge to differentiate the effects of dietary fat on lipoproteins and cardiovascular disease risk in men and women, in the different lipid disorders, and in the metabolic syndrome.

14. Protective nutrients and functional foods for the gastrointestinal tract. Christopher Duggan, Jennifer Gannon and W Allan Walker. American *Journal of Clinical Nutrition*, Vol. 75, No. 5, 789-808, May 2002.

The term functional food is used to describe nutrients that have an effect on physiologic processes that is separate from their established nutritional function, and some of these nutrients are proposed to promote gastrointestinal mucosal integrity. We reviewed the recent in vitro, animal, and clinical experiments that evaluated the role of several types of gastrointestinal functional foods, including the amino acids glutamine and arginine, the essential micronutrients vitamin A and zinc, and 2 classes of food additives, prebiotics and probiotics.

15. Infant vision and retinal function in studies of dietary long-chain polyunsaturated fatty acids: methods, results, and implications. Martha Neuringer. *American Journal of Clinical Nutrition*, Vol. 71, No. 1, 256-267, January 2000.

Animal and human studies have documented several effects of different dietary and tissue concentrations of long-chain polyunsaturated fatty acids (LCPUFAs) on retinal function and vision. The enhanced visual development associated with increased intakes of LCPUFAs, particularly docosahexaenoic acid (DHA), provides the strongest evidence for the importance of these fatty acids in infant nutrition.

16. Dietary fats, carbohydrates, and progression of coronary atherosclerosis in postmenopausal women. Dariush Mozaffarian, Eric B Rimm and David M Herrington. *American Journal of Clinical Nutrition*, Vol. 80, No. 5, 1175-1184, November 2004.

In postmenopausal women with relatively low total fat intake, a greater saturated-fat intake is associated with less progression of coronary atherosclerosis, whereas carbohydrate intake is associated with a greater progression.

17. Yogurt and gut function. Oskar Adolfsson, Simin Nikbin Meydani and Robert M Russell. *American Journal of Clinical Nutrition*, Vol. 80, No. 2, 245-256, August 2004.

It has long been believed that the consumption of yogurt and other fermented milk products provides various health benefits. Recent studies of the possible health benefits of yogurt in gut-associated diseases substantiate some of these beliefs. Of particular interest are the reduction—by yogurt, yogurt bacteria, or both—in the duration of diarrheal diseases in children, the preventive or therapeutic (or both) effects on IBD and colon cancer as suggested by epidemiologic evidence and animal studies, and the possible beneficial effects in increasing the eradication rate of H. pylori as indicated by in vitro and preliminary human studies. In addition, there is ever-increasing evidence of the beneficial effect of yogurt containing live and active cultures on the digestion of lactose in persons with lactose intolerance.

18. Prebiotics and probiotics: are they functional foods? Marcel B Roberfroid *American Journal of Clinical Nutrition*, Vol. 71, No. 6, 1682S-1687s, June 2000.

These products favorably influence digestive functions and colonic flora. The most promising health benefits are the prevention of diarrhea and enhancement of the immune system.

19. Dietary and other risk factors for stroke in Hawaiian Japanese men. A Kagan, JS Popper, GG Rhoads and K Yano, *Stroke*, Vol 16, 390-396

In this study, no relation was found between salt intake and the incidence of stroke.

20. Effects of a ketogenic diet on tumor metabolism and nutritional status in pediatric oncology patients: two case reports. L. C. Nebeling, F. Miraldi, S. B. Shurin and E. Lerner, Journal of the *American College of Nutrition*, Vol 14, Issue 2 202-208.

Within 7 days of initiating the ketogenic diet, blood glucose levels declined to low-normal levels and blood ketones were elevated twenty to thirty fold. Results of PET scans indicated a 21.8% average decrease in glucose uptake at the tumor site in both subjects. One patient exhibited significant clinical improvements in mood and new skill development during the study. She continued the ketogenic diet for an additional twelve months, remaining free of disease progression. While this diet does not replace conventional antineoplastic treatments, these preliminary results suggest a potential for clinical application which merits further research.

21. Vitamin D, Calcium and Prevention of Breast Cancer: A Review. Martin Lipkin, MD and Harold L. Newmark, DSc, *Journal of the American College of Nutrition*, Vol. 18, No. 90005, 392S-397S (1999).

Reduction of breast cancer risk, simultaneously with several other cancers and with osteoporosis, might be achieved by increasing the dietary intake of vitamin D and calcium to current recommended levels.

22. Benefits of Dairy Product Consumption on Blood Pressure in Humans: A Summary of the Biomedical Literature. Gregory D. Miller, PhD, Douglas D. DiRienzo, PhD, Molly E. Reusser, BA and David A. McCarron, MD , *Journal of the American College of Nutrition*, Vol. 19, No. 90002, 147S-164S (2000).

FYI: Thirty-one studies have shown that low blood cholesterol correlates with higher cancer or total death rates.

After two decades of intense clinical investigation this study yielded consistent, reproducible evidence from epidemiologic surveys and randomized control trials that consumption of dairy products decreases the risk of hypertensive heart disease and may optimize arterial pressure control.

23. The Effects of Varying Dietary Fat on the Nutrient Intake in Male and Female Runners. Peter J. Horvath, PhD, FACN, CNS, Colleen K. Eagen, MS, Stacie D. Ryer-Calvin, BA and David R. Pendergast, EdD, *Journal of the American College of Nutrition*, Vol. 19, No. 1, 42-51 (2000).

    In summary, adequate caloric intake and proper nutrition are important for the optimal performance and health of athletes. We can conclude from our data that on a low fat diet it was not possible for these runners to consume the recommended levels of all the RDAs or the required amount of calories.

24. The Importance of Meeting Calcium Needs with Foods. Gregory D. Miller, PhD, FACN, Judith K. Jarvis, MS, RD, LD and Lois D. McBean, MS, RD *Journal of the American College of Nutrition*, Vol. 20, No. 2, 168S-185S (2001).

    Foods are the preferred source of calcium. Milk and other dairy foods are the major source of calcium in the U.S. In addition, these foods provide substantial amounts of other essential nutrients. Consequently, intake of dairy foods improves the overall nutritional quality of the diet.

25. The Role of Calcium In Prevention of Chronic Diseases. Gregory D. Miller, PhD and John J.B. Anderson, PhD, *Journal of the American College of Nutrition*, Vol. 18, No. 90005, 371S-372S (1999)

    Calcium is involved in reducing the risk of osteoporosis, hypertension, colon cancer, breast cancer, kidney stones, and lead intoxication.

26. Dairy Foods and Prevention of Colon Cancer: Human Studies. Peter R. Holt, MD, *Journal of the American College of Nutrition*, Vol. 18, No. 90005, 379S-391S (1999).

    International and national incidence rates for colon cancer suggest an inverse relationship with dietary calcium and/or vitamin D intake (or sun exposure).

27. Low plasma vitamin B-6 concentrations and modulation of coronary artery disease risk. Simonetta Friso, Domenico Girelli, Nicola Martinelli, Oliviero Olivieri, Valentina Lotto, Claudia Bozzini, Francesca Pizzolo, Giovanni Faccini, Federico Beltrame, and Roberto Corrocher.

    Low plasma PLP concentrations are inversely related to major markers of inflammation and independently associated with increased CAD risk.

28. Calcium, vitamin D, and the occurrence of colorectal cancer among women. ME Martinez, EL Giovannucci, GA Colditz, MJ Stampfer, DJ Hunter, FE Speizer, A Wing and WC Willett, *Journal Of The National Cancer Institute*, Vol 88, 1375-1382.

These findings do not support a substantial inverse association between calcium intake and risk of colorectal cancer, but an inverse association between intake of total vitamin D and risk of colorectal cancer was suggested.

29. Calcium, Vitamin D, and Risk for Colorectal Adenoma Dependency on Vitamin D Receptor BsmI Polymorphism and Nonsteroidal Anti-Inflammatory Drug Use. Sonia M. Boyapati, Roberd M. Bostick, Katherine A. McGlynn, Michael F. Fina, Walter M. Roufail, Kim R. Geisinger, Michael Wargovich, Ann Coker and James R. Hebert, *Cancer Epidemiology Biomarkers and Prevention* Vol. 12, 631-637, July 2003.

In summary, our findings of modest, inverse associations of increasing calcium and vitamin D intakes and risk for colorectal adenoma are similar to those estimates reported in previous observational epidemiological studies.

30. Calcium Intake and Risk of Colon Cancer in Women and Men. Kana Wu, Walter C. Willett, Charles S. Fuchs, Graham A. Colditz, Edward L. Giovannucci, *Journal of the National Cancer Institute,* Vol. 94, No. 6, 437-446, March 20, 2002.

Our results suggest that relatively moderate calcium intake may decrease the risk of distal colon cancer but that high calcium intake may not appreciably lower the risk further. Considering the public health importance of colon cancer, even a modest protective effect of higher calcium intake on colon cancer could result in the prevention of a large number of colon cancer cases.

31. RESPONSE: Re: Calcium Intake and Risk of Colon Cancer in Women and Men. Kana Wu, Edward L. Giovannucci, *Journal of the National Cancer Institute*, Vol. 95, No. 2, 169-170, January 15, 2003

We concur that increasing calcium intake for some individuals may have an important role in the prevention of distal colon cancer.

32. Assessment of dietary vitamin D requirements during pregnancy and lactation. Bruce W Hollis and Carol L Wagner, *American Journal of Clinical Nutrition*, Vol. 79, No. 5, 717-726, May 2004.

We believe that it is time to reexamine the understated DRI of vitamin D for lactating mothers.

33. Chronic sunscreen use decreases circulating concentrations of 25-hydroxyvitamin D. A preliminary stud. L. Y. Matsuoka, J. Wortsman, N. Hanifan and M. F. Holick, *Archives of Dermatology*, Vol. 124, No. 12, December 1988.

This preliminary study suggests that long-term use of PABA may be associated with low body stores of vitamin D in some persons. Letters.

34. Vitamin D concentrations in Asian children living in England. Stanley Zlotkin, Professor. *BMJ* 1999;318:1417 (22 May)

FYI: The average blood cholesterol is 220 mg. Since the current guideline for high cholesterol is 200 mg., most of the population is classified as high. Cholesterol treatment and testing is one of the most lucrative industries in the world.

With the increasing use of sunscreen one may justifiably ask whether infants and children are at an increased risk of vitamin D deficiency.

35. Abnormal T-cell subset proportions in vitamin-A-deficient children. Semba RD, Muhilal, Ward BJ, Griffin DE, Scott AL, Natadisastra G, West KP Jr, Sommer A., *Lancet*. 1993 Jan 2;341(8836):5-8.

Vitamin-A-deficient children have underlying immune abnormalities in T-cell subsets and these abnormalities are reversible with vitamin A supplementation.

36. Lymphocyte Development and Function in the Absence of Retinoic Acid-Related Orphan Receptor. Ivan Dzhagalov, Vincent Giguère and You-Wen He, *The Journal of Immunology*, 2004, 173: 2952-2959.

These results indicate that RORα indirectly regulates lymphocyte development by providing an appropriate microenvironment and controls immune responses by negatively regulating cytokine production in innate immune cells and lymphocytes.

37. Evidence for potential mechanisms for the effect of conjugated linoleic acid on tumor metabolism and immune function: lessons from n–3 fatty acids. Catherine J Field and Patricia D Schley, *American Journal of Clinical Nutrition*, Vol. 79, No. 6, 1190S-1198S, June 2004.

Conjugated linoleic acid (CLA) and the long-chain polyunsaturated n–3 fatty acids have been shown in vivo and in vitro to reduce tumor growth.

38. Immunomodulatory properties of conjugated linoleic acid. Marianne O'Shea, Josep Bassaganya-Riera and Inge CM Mohede, *American Journal of Clinical Nutrition*, Vol. 79, No. 6, 1199S-1206S, June 2004.

The understanding of the mechanism(s) by which CLA increases immune function will aid in the development of nutritionally based therapeutic applications to augment host resistance against infectious diseases and to treat immune imbalances, which result in inflammatory disorders, allergic reactions, or both.

39. Association of Dietary Intake of Fat and Fatty Acids With Risk of Breast Cancer. Michelle D. Holmes, MD, DrPH; David J. Hunter, MB, BS, ScD; Graham A. Colditz, MD, DrPH; Meir J. Stampfer, MD, DrPH; Susan E. Hankinson, ScD; Frank E. Speizer, MD; Bernard Rosner, PhD; Walter C. Willett, MD, DrPH, *JAMA*. 1999;281:914-920.

We found no evidence that lower intake of total fat or specific major types of fat was associated with a decreased risk of breast cancer.

40. Carbohydrates and the Risk of Breast Cancer among Mexican Women. Isabelle Romieu, Eduardo Lazcano-Ponce, Luisa Maria Sanchez-Zamorano, Walter Willett and Mauricio Hernandez-Avila *Cancer Epidemiology Biomarkers and Prevention* Vol. 13, 1283-1289, August 2004.

In this population-based case-control study, we observed a positive association between carbohydrate intake and the risk of breast cancer.

41. Effects of low-fat, high-carbohydrate diets on risk factors for ischemic heart disease in postmenopausal women [published erratum appears in Am J Clin Nutr 1997 Aug; 66(2):437], J Jeppesen, P Schaaf, C Jones, MY Zhou, YD Chen and GM Reaven, *American Journal of Clinical Nutrition*, Vol 65, 1027-1033.

Because all of these changes would increase risk of ischemic heart disease in postmenopausal women, it seems reasonable to question the wisdom of recommending that postmenopausal women consume low-fat, high-carbohydrate diets.

42. Dairy Consumption, Obesity, and the Insulin Resistance Syndrome in Young Adults. The CARDIA Study, Mark A. Pereira, PhD; David R. Jacobs, Jr, PhD; Linda Van Horn, PhD,RD; Martha L. Slattery, PhD,RD; Alex I. Kartashov, PhD; David S. Ludwig, MD,PhD, *JAMA*. 2002;287:2081-2089.

Dietary patterns characterized by increased dairy consumption have a strong inverse association with IRS among overweight adults and may reduce risk of type 2 diabetes and cardiovascular disease.

43. Consumption of dairy products and the risk of breast cancer: a review of the literature. Patricia G Moorman and Paul D Terry, *American Journal of Clinical Nutrition*, Vol. 80, No. 1, 5-14, July 2004

The available epidemiologic evidence does not support a strong association between the consumption of milk or other dairy products and breast cancer risk.

44. Role of calcium and dairy products in energy partitioning and weight management. Michael B Zemel, *American Journal of Clinical Nutrition*, Vol. 79, No. 5, 907S-912S, May 2004

These data indicate an important role for dairy products in both the prevention and treatment of obesity.

45. Consumption of fermented and nonfermented dairy products: effects on cholesterol concentrations and metabolism. Marie-Pierre St-Onge, Edward R Farnworth and Peter JH Jones, *American Journal of Clinical Nutrition*, Vol. 71, No. 3, 674-681, March 2000

In light of these findings, several fermented dairy products available on the market today have the potential of being classified as useful cholesterol-lowering agents. These foods include fermented vegetables, bifidus- and acidophilus-containing yogurt and milk beverages, and kefir, a fermented dairy product containing several types of bacteria in symbiosis with yeasts.

FYI: Polyunsaturated oils that are hydrogenated cause cholesterol levels to rise, yet they are advertised as "heart protection." An example is margarine that contains a large amount of trans-fatty acids that are produced when polyunsaturated oils are hydrogenated.

46. Dietary fat and obesity: an epidemiologic perspective. JC Seidell, *American Journal of Clinical Nutrition*, Vol. 67, 546S-550S, Copyright © 1998.

   The observation that dietary fat has an effect on weight gain and the development of obesity that is larger than would be expected on the basis of fat's energy value is mainly experimental. At this stage there is no conclusive evidence from epidemiologic studies that under isoenergetic conditions dietary fat intake promotes the development of obesity more so than other macronutrients.

47. A Reduced Ratio of Dietary Carbohydrate to Protein Improves Body Composition and Blood Lipid Profiles during Weight Loss in Adult Women. Donald K. Layman, Richard A. Boileau, Donna J. Erickson, James E. Painter, Harn Shiue, Carl Sather, and Demtra D. Christou· J. *Nutr.* 133:411-417, February 2003

   This study demonstrates that increasing the proportion of protein to carbohydrate in the diet of adult women has positive effects on body composition, blood lipids, glucose homeostasis and satiety during weight loss.

48. Dietary protein and risk of ischemic heart disease in women. Frank B Hu, Meir J Stampfer, JoAnn E Manson, Eric Rimm, Graham A Colditz, Frank E Speizer, Charles H Hennekens and Walter C Willett, *American Journal of Clinical Nutrition*, Vol. 70, No. 2, 221-227, August 1999.

   Our data do not support the hypothesis that a high protein intake increases the risk of ischemic heart disease. In contrast, our findings suggest that replacing carbohydrates with protein may be associated with a lower risk of ischemic heart disease. Because a high dietary protein intake is often accompanied by increases in saturated fat and cholesterol intakes, application of these findings to public dietary advice should be cautious.

49. Short-term effects of substituting protein for carbohydrate in the diets of moderately hypercholesterolemic human subjects. Wolfe BM, Giovannetti PM., *Metabolism.* 1991 Apr; 40(4):338-43.

   The short-term effects on plasma lipoprotein lipids of substituting meat and dairy protein for carbohydrate in the diets of 10 free-living moderately hypercholesterolemic human subjects (four men, six women) were studied under closely supervised dietary control during the consumption of constant, low intakes of fat and cholesterol and the maintenance of stable body weight as well as constant fiber consumption.

50. Effect of a High-Protein, High–Monounsaturated Fat Weight Loss Diet on Glycemic Control and Lipid Levels in Type 2 Diabetes. Barbara Parker, BSC, Manny Noakes, PHD, Natalie Luscombe, BSC, and Peter Clifton, MD, PHD, *Diabetes Care* 25:425-430, 2002

The greater reductions in total and abdominal fat mass in women and greater LDL cholesterol reduction observed in both sexes on the HP diet suggest that it is a valid diet choice for reducing CVD risk in type-2 diabetes.

51. Daily methionine requirements of healthy Indian men, measured by a 24-h indicator amino acid oxidation and balance technique. Anura V Kurpad, Meredith M Regan, Sureka Varalakshmi, Jahnavi Vasudevan, Justin Gnanou, Tony Raj and Vernon R Young, *American Journal of Clinical Nutrition*, Vol. 77, No. 5, 1198-1205, May 2003

    In summary, the present investigation of 24-h [^{13}C] leucine tracer indicator kinetics in well-nourished Indian subjects studied with 7 test intakes of methionine, including the 1985 FAO/WHO/UNU SAA requirement of 13 mg • kg^{-1} • d^{-1}, indicates that the international mean requirement for total SAAs (specifically, methionine in the absence of a dietary cystine source) should be close to 15 mg • kg^{-1} • d^{-1}.

52. Total sulfur amino acid requirement in young men as determined by indicator amino acid oxidation with L-[1-^{13}C] phenylalanine. Marco Di Buono, Linda J Wykes, Ronald O Ball, and Paul B Pencharz, *American Journal of Clinical Nutrition*, Vol. 74, No. 6, 756-760, December 2001

    Although the mean SAA requirement is consistent with current guidelines for the total SAA intake, the population-safe intake is substantially higher than the currently recommended total SAA intake.

53. Recent advances in methods of assessing dietary amino acid requirements for adult humans. Zello GA, Wykes LJ, Ball RO, Pencharz PB., *J Nutr*. 1995 Dec; 125(12):2907-15.

    The requirements for the indispensable amino acids have been determined by a number of different methods. Historically, descriptive or gross measures like growth and nitrogen balance have been used. However, technological advancements in recent years have resulted in the use of more precise and mechanistic metabolic approaches (i.e., plasma amino acid concentrations, amino acid oxidation, indicator amino acid oxidation) to examine requirement. Nevertheless, the current recommendations are still based on nitrogen balance studies. Requirement estimates based on other methodologies, such as plasma amino acid concentrations and direct amino acid oxidation, suggest that the requirement estimates derived from nitrogen balance experiments are too low.

54. Tryptophan requirement in young adult women as determined by indicator amino acid oxidation with L-[13C] phenylalanine. G Lazaris-Brunner, M Rafii, RO Ball and PB Pencharz, *American Journal of Clinical Nutrition*, Vol 68, 303-310, Copyright © 1998.

    Our value of safe intake for 95% of the population was found to be 43% higher than that reported previously for adults.

55. Phase of menstrual cycle affects lysine requirement in healthy women, *Am J Physiol Endocrinol Metab* 287: E489-E496, 2004, Wantanee Kriengsinyos, Linda J. Wykes, Laksiri A. Goonewardene, Ronald O. Ball, and Paul B. Pencharz.

Therefore, we reason that the higher lysine requirement observed in the luteal phase is probably due to higher amino acid catabolism.

56. What Are the Essential Elements Needed for the Determination of Amino Acid Requirements in Humans? Peter Fürst and Peter Stehle, *J. Nutr.* 134:1558S-1565S, June 2004.

Despite important achievements, many problems still remain to be solved concerning the requirements of specific amino acids before the nutritional treatment of wasting diseases can be optimized. Current results of metabolic studies indicate that the composition, amounts, and proportions of the presently available nutritional preparations are not suitable for the treatment of critically or chronically ill catabolic patients.

57. 1,25-Dihydroxycholecalciferol Prevents and Ameliorates Symptoms of Experimental Murine Inflammatory Bowel Disease. Margherita T. Cantorna, Carey Munsick, Candace Bemiss and Brett D. Mahon, *Journal of Nutrition.* 2000;130:2648-2652.

The results suggest that plant foods may be important in the etiology of rectal cancer in both men and women.

58. Vitamin D: importance in the prevention of cancers, type 1 diabetes, heart disease, and osteoporosis. Michael F Holick, *American Journal of Clinical Nutrition*, Vol. 79, No. 3, 362-371, March 2004

Anecdotal data suggest that the amount of vitamin D available in the environment either from sunshine exposure or diet may be an important factor affecting the development of inflammatory bowel disease (IBD) in humans.

Studies in both human and animal models add strength to the hypothesis that the unrecognized epidemic of vitamin D deficiency worldwide is a contributing factor of many chronic debilitating diseases. Greater awareness of the insidious consequences of vitamin D deficiency is needed. Annual measurement of serum 25(OH) D is a reasonable approach to monitoring for vitamin D deficiency. The recommended adequate intakes for vitamin D are inadequate, and, in the absence of exposure to sunlight, a minimum of 1000 IU vitamin D/d is required to maintain a healthy concentration of 25(OH) D in the blood.

59. Plant foods, fiber, and rectal cancer. Martha L Slattery, Karen P Curtin, Sandra L Edwards and Donna M Schaffer, *American Journal of Clinical Nutrition*, Vol. 79, No. 2, 274-281, February 2004.

FYI: The Chinese diet contains very little milk, meat, and eggs. They also have a high rate of atherosclerosis.

RECOMMENDED READING

Nutrition and Physical Degeneration by Weston A Price 6th edition, 14th printing. La Mesa, CA, USA. Price-Pottenger Nutrition Foundation, 2000. This is the book promoted by the Weston A. Price Foundation. Everybody and anybody who is interested in nutrition, or who has an opinion on nutrition, must read this enduring classic. This book was researched when it was still possible to compare groups of people living on a traditional diet to those people of the same racial stock living on the foods of commerce (Western diet).

Nourishing Traditions; The Cookbook that Challenges Politically Correct Nutrition and the Diet Dictocrats by Sally Fallon, New Trends Publishing, Inc. Washington, DC. This book provides high-quality information on traditional foods that builds upon the work of Dr Weston A. Price. It is has hundreds of recipes based on the diets of traditional peoples.

The Metabolic Typing Diet Book by William Wolcott and Trish Fahey, Broadway Books, New York, NY. With this book, you can customize your diet to your own unique body chemistry. The writers provide simple self-tests that you can use to discover your own metabolic type and determine what kind of diet will work best for you.

Biochemical Individuality by Roger J. Williams, Keats Publishing, New Canaan, CT. A timeless classic that links the diversity in our anatomy and body chemistry to our unique nutritional needs.

The Untold Story of Milk by Ron Schmid After intense research and interviews with farmers across the country, Dr. Ron Schmid brings us a definitive new book on the history, benefits, and future of raw milk! Chapters include: Milk in Early America, The Distillery Dairies, History of the Milk Cure, Betrayal by Health Officials, Safety and Health Benefits of Raw Milk.

Raw Milk Source Guide by Redemske Design, 833 Colrain Rd, Greenfield, MA 01301. E-mail Sandy Redemske atsandyr@shaysnet.com. Includes: the supplemental report in favor of raw milk; milk cures many diseases; health benefits of raw milk from grass-fed animals; why butter is better; the case for butter; fermented milk; raising healthy dairy cows; traditional cultures and raw milk; resources.

The Fourfold Path of Healing by Thomas Cowan, M.D with Sally Fallon and Jaimen McMillan. New Trends Publishing, Inc. Washington, DC 20007 Copyright 2004.

FYI: Cholesterol does not cause heart disease. Sally Fallon and her co-author Dr. Mary Enig have written a Four-part series called "The Oiling of America." Sally has presented this powerful story at live events around the country and it is also available on the Web at: www.westonaprice.org/knowyourfats/oiling.html.

The Cholesterol Myths by Uffe Ravnskov, MD, Ph D. Did you know that cholesterol is not a deadly poison, but a substance vital to the cells of all mammals? Dr. Ravnskov exposes the faulty premises and questionable science behind the diet-heart idea. Before you adopt a low-fat diet or take expensive cholesterol-lowering drugs, read his excellent analysis in The Cholesterol Myths.

The Second Brain by Michael D. Gershon, M.D., HarperCollins Publishers, Inc. New York, NY., Dr. Michael Gershon has devoted his career to understanding the human bowels (the stomach, esophagus, small intestine, and colon). His thirty years of research have led to an extraordinary rediscovery: nerve cells in the gut that act as a brain.

Nutrition and Your Mind: The Psychochemical Response by George Watson. Watson published this book in 1972. As a founding father of psychochemistry, he clearly details his perspective that most mental-health issues can readily be resolved through balancing body biochemistry. Using clinical case histories, he presents important principles that he has uncovered over a twenty-year period.

Pottenger's Cats - a Study in Nutrition by Francis M. Pottenger, Jr., MD. A comparison of healthy cats on raw foods and those on heated diets. Behavioral characteristics, arthritis, sterility, skeletal deformities and, allergies are some of the problems that are associated with the consumption of cooked foods.

Sugar Blues by William Dufty, Warner Books, 1975. When cultures first had access to sugar on a commercial scale, they probably reacted to it the same way that our modern cultures have reacted to heroin and cocaine. Unfortunately, we have all become so accustomed to our daily fix of sugar that few people are even prepared to conduct an experiment and totally eliminate refined sugar from their diet for even one day.

Body Ecology Diet: Recovering Your Health and Rebuilding Your Immunity, by Donna Gates, B.E.D Publications, 1996, This book gives an added perspective to Ten Days as it shows you how to restore and maintain the inner ecology your body needs to function properly and to eliminate or control the symptoms of candidiasis.

The Maker's Diet by Jordan Rubin

Wild Fermentation by Sandor Ellix Katz

Know Your Fats: The Complete Primer for Understanding the Nutrition of Fats, Oils and Cholesterol by Mary Enig

Facts About Fats, A Consumer's Guide to Good Oils, John Finnegan Published: 1993, Publisher: Celestial Arts. This book explains the body's need for fatty acids, recommends the most healthful oils, and discusses weight management.

The Milk Book, by Dr. William Campbell Douglas. Once upon a time, raw milk was what people drank in the U.S., and it sustained generations of healthy people. Learn about the wonderful benefits of certified raw milk, the harmful effects of pasteurized milk, and the eye-opening story of how we got from here to there. A classic.

We Want to Live, Aajonus Vonderplanitz, Carnelian Bay Castle Press, LLC, 1997.

The Pulse Test: The Secret of Building Your Basic Health
by Arthur F. Coca, M.D.. Allergies? This book shows you how to find your personal food and inhalant allergies, and how to avoid them using your pulse., Barricade Books, Inc., New York, NY.10003, 1994.

FYI: Americans consume 500 times more vegetable fat than they did in 1920.

FYI: Check your local library for the following video (Video cassette or DVD):

Sweet Misery
Sound and Fury
Productions 2004

FYI: Doctors do not study nutrition in medical school.

INDEX

FYI: Doctors are trained to treat illness with drugs.

FYI: By limiting cholesterol in our diets, we risk getting sick with serious generative disease.

FYI: The American Heart Association has been promoting a low-cholesterol diet since 1961 and ignores studies that say there is no relationship between diet and coronary heart disease.

FYI: Homocysteine is considered to be a strong independent risk factor for heat disease.

Genome 14
GERD 65
Gerson cancer treatment 59
Gerson, Dr. Max 59, 138
Giardia 124
Glass 33, 46, 92, 93, 97, 98, 100. 140, 148, 185, 187
Glucocorticoids 37
Glutathione S-Transferase (GST) 139
Glycemic Index (GI) 75
Glycerin enema 145
Goats 6, 45, 68
Goitrogens 5
Grains 1, 19, 29, 39, 58, 68, 71, 72, 73, 74, 75, 98, 99, 137, 150, 153
Grass-fed butter 10, 25, 47, 144, 151
Grass-fed meat 25, 15, 45
Greeks 8, 56, 60
Green tea enema 145

G

Hair analysis 91, 119
Harrill, Rex 54, 55, 56, 57
HDL cholesterol 54, 164
Healing crisis 9
Health and Healing Wisdom 16
Health meats 45
Healthexcel ii
Healthy Baby Gallery 100
Healthy fats 25, 28, 47
Healthy soil environment viii
Healthy vs. unhealthy fats 27
Healy, Dr. Bernadette 164
Heart disease 42, 49
Heavy metals 10, 26. 83, 91, 92
Hemorrhoids 70, 145, 147
Herbal teas 96
Here on Earth 5
High blood pressure 8, 49, 63, 70, 72
High enema 142

FYI: If your doctor is not familar with homocysteine and you would like yours checked, contact the Life Extension Foundation (www.lef.org). They will refer you to a blood lab that can offer a test and help you interpret the results.

Kefir grains 39, 98, 137
Kefir-making e-group 121
Kelley, Dr. William Donald 138
Kenueke, Robin 58
Kingsolver, Barbara 1
Kombucha 37, 70, 76, 80, 84, 85, 86, 89, 93, 99, 100, 101, 102, 103, 153, 154, 155
Kombucha scobies 74
Kvass 19, 26, 56, 71, 89, 93, 97, 103
KY Jelly 134

L
Lacto-fermented foods 19, 26, 56, 97, 98, 99, 168
Lactoperoxidase 75
Lactose 46, 61, 68, 99
Lavender 60, 61, 133, 147
LDL cholesterol 50
Leaky gut 64, 74, 115
Licorice root 146
Lipase 11, 48, 60, 68, 77
Lipitor 77
Liver 1, 11, 25, 32, 37, 40, 43, 46, 48, 50, 52, 57, 59, 63, 78, 87, 97, 104, 115
Liver, raw 52
Living Fuel 94, 103, 150, 154
Living the Good Life 14
Livingston-Wheeler, Virginia 45
Localharvest.org 2, 29
Low-fat diet 53, 56, 78
Low-fat milk 162
Lungs 9, 32, 83
Lymphatic systems 9

M
Maasai 156
Mad Cow Disease 45, 59, 109
Magnesium 154
Magnetic clay baths 91
Maori 18

FYI: The medical commnunity refuses to acknowledge the homocysteine theory.

FYI: When polyunsaturated oils are heated, they form peroxides that are toxic.

Raw meat 46, 47, 59
Raw milk 3, 15, 59, 69, 75, 79, 81, 83, 91, 94, 95, 102, 103, 104, 120, 121, 135
Raw milk and molasses enema 148
Realmilk.com 91, 94, 95, 111
Reclaiming Our Health 149
Re-evaluation Counseling ii
Riboflavin 7
Robbins, John 149
Robinson, Jo 67
Romans 8, 60

S
Safe fish 25, 45
Salmonella Infections 81, 131
Saturated fats 19, 28, 49, 56, 58, 157, 160
Sauerkraut 61, 62, 68, 69
Schmid, Dr. Ron 98, 131
Schuld, Andreas 126
Schizophrenia 42, 100
Scoby 37, 101, 102, 103
Second brain, 124
Second Brain, The 170
Sesame oil 29, 53, 125, 146, 156
Sexual steroidal hormones 37
Shaw, George Bernard 137
Shell fish 48
Sigmoid colon 113, 130, 134, 135, 140, 144
Skin 9, 32, 50, 59, 60, 63, 65, 70, 71, 118
Sleep 34, 40, 69, 74, 150, 151
Slippery elm bark 145
Slippery elm enema 145
Slow Food Movement 16
Small meals 25, 36
Soda 73, 80, 81, 152
Soups 26, 62, 63, 95, 97
Soy foods 43, 62, 70, 71, 89, 90, 92, 137, 149
Soy Online Service 82
Springsteen, Bruce 7

FYI: Cheesecloth provides a fine mesh to strain your kombucha. Use one layer and secure it to a wide-mouth glass container with a rubber band.

U

U.S. Department of Agriculture, 18, 145
Untold Story of Milk, The 98, 131,
USDA food pyramid 58

V

Vegetable fat 1, 171
Vegetable juice 10, 40, 59, 91, 95, 103, 104, 106
Vegetable juicer 40
Vita Mix 40, 95, 96
Vitamin A 9, 19, 48, 50, 65, 66, 152
Vitamin B12 36, 42
Vitamin B6 100
Vitamin C and the Common Cold 14
Vitamin D 9, 19, 43, 48, 50, 63, 65, 68
Vitamin E 52
Vit-Ra-Tox 106
Vit-Ra-Tox supplements 96

W

Washburn, Lindy 20
Water 24, 32, 34, 125, 126, 130, 131, 132, 133, 134, 136, 140, 141, 142, 143, 144, 145, 146, 150
Water, municipal 124
Water-kefir 39
Weber State University 147
Weil, Dr. Andrew 16
Weston A. Price Foundation iii, 104, 105
Weston A. Price Foundation Chapter, Madison 3
Weston A. Price Foundation Web site 110
Weston A. Price Foundation, local chapters 142
Wheat Germ/Flax Oil 106, 107
Wheat grass enema 144
White Egret Farms 70, 79, 81, 83, 95
Whole Soy Story, The 89
Wilderness Family Naturals 94
Wisconsin Public Radio 5
Wise Traditions Magazine 54, 55, 57, 143
Wulzen factor 28, 64

FYI: Because the glucoronic acid in kombucha will pull plastic into your kombucha, glass is the best material for bottling it. It is important that the bottle does not have a metal cap. Juice bottles sold at health-food stores have lids that are lined, and they may be recycled for storing kombucha. At room temperature, gas will accumulate in a closed container. If you leave your kombucha out of the refrigerator and you don't drink it right away, you will need to release the gas that accumulates. Always open kombucha bottles carefully, in case there is a gas build-up.

FYI: The message board on www.optimalhealth-network.com includes an active network of people who support each other by sharing their stories about how colon cleansing improved their health. Please do take some time to ready through the many posts.

CPSIA information can be obtained at www.ICGtesting.com
263768BV00003B/73/A